Advance Praise for *Islamically Integrated Psychotherapy*

"Al-Karam has assembled a diverse and talented team to demonstrate how psychology (and psychotherapy in particular) can be approached from a Muslim worldview. This remarkable and nuanced work will serve the field by spurring discussion, promoting understanding, and hopefully igniting research in the area. I heartily encourage it as a starting point for all who want to understand and work effectively with Muslims in therapy."

— TIM SISEMORE, PhD, president of APA's Society for the Psychology of Religion and Spirituality (Div. 36) and author of *The Psychology of Religion and Spirituality: From the Inside Out* (Wiley)

"This edited volume makes a profound contribution to the existing literature on psychotherapy broadly, and amplifies the voices of Muslim practitioners. Among the most salient features are the diverse treatment modalities featured, the weaving of conceptual and practical content, and the range of audiences that can benefit from the book!"

— ALTAF HUSAIN, MSSA, PhD, associate professor, Howard University School of Social Work and vice president, Yaqeen Institute for Islamic Research

"The book is a testimony to the profound multifaceted contributions of a new generation of Muslim psychologists. Just by reading the titles of the chapters and the names of the authors, any psychologist practicing in the Muslim world would find it necessary to have it as a reference for helping him or her with the unique problems of Muslim clients."

— MALIK BADRI, professor of Psychology, Istanbul Zaim University

"This is a timely book to guide practitioners worldwide in developing and using Islamic paradigms and principles in their work. The need to share their insights is paramount in taking this field further to the Muslim community and to the mainstream globally."
> —NASIMA KHANOM, Consultant Specialist Systemic/Family Psychotherapist and founding chair of the Islamic Psychology Professional Association (IPPA)

"A timely, bold and much-needed work offering insights into working with Muslim clients all over the world."
> —AMBER HAQUE, PhD, professor of Clinical Psychology, United Arab Emirates University

"This book is a landmark in the epiphany of Islamic Psychology in the West: a 'must read' for all those with an interest in the field."
> —RASJID SKINNER, consultant clinical psychologist and visiting professor of Clinical Psychology at the University of Karachi

"Carrie York Al-Karam has edited a must-read primer for any counselor or therapist working with Muslim patients and couples. After reading this book, you will have learned from some of the best researchers in the field."
> —RUKHSANA M. CHAUDHRY PsyD, director of Mental Health Programming, American Muslim Health Professionals

"This is a remarkable and skillfully written book. All the chapters give us the opportunity to explore and better understand psychology through the Islamic lens. I applaud this initiative, and highly recommend this book to be a source of reference for all in the field of psychology."
> —JOANNE HANDS, PhD, LPC, LMFT, president, Middle East Psychological Association

Islamically Integrated
Psychotherapy

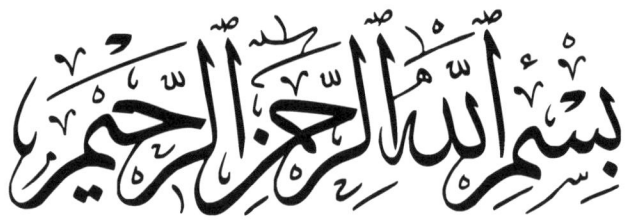

Bismillah al-Rahman al-Raheem

In the name of God, the most Gracious, the most Merciful

ISLAMICALLY
INTEGRATED
PSYCHOTHERAPY

Uniting Faith and Professional Practice

EDITED BY

Carrie York Al-Karam, PhD

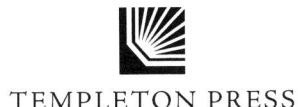

TEMPLETON PRESS

Templeton Press
300 Conshohocken State Road, Suite 500
West Conshohocken, PA 19428
www.templetonpress.org

Set in Adobe Jenson pro by Gopa & Ted2, Inc.

Library of Congress Control Number: 2018943026
ISBN: 978-1-59947-581-3 (pbk: alk. paper)
eISBN: 978-1-59947-542-4

This paper meets the requirements of ANSI/NISO Z39.48-1992
(Permanence of Paper).
A catalogue record for this book is available
from the Library of Congress.

20 21 22 23 24   10 9 8 7 6 5 4 3 2 1

Printed in the United States of America.

Contents

This book is dedicated to the
global Muslim community.

Acknowledgments

GETTING A BOOK published is like raising a child—it literally takes a village! Much thanks is owed to so many people who contributed to the successful completion of this edited volume. I am grateful to be able to thank them in this public space.

I'd like to first thank the John Templeton Foundation for its support of this work. It is an incredible honor to be associated with this wonderful organization. Regarding this project specifically, endless thanks are directed to Templeton Press and the tireless efforts by the individuals who work hard there every day to make such publications come to fruition: Susan Arellano, publisher; Angelina Horst, senior publishing coordinator; Daniel Reilly, marketing and publicity coordinator, and Trish Vergilio, production and design coordinator. Many thanks to this amazing team!

Of course this book simply would not exist without the generous contribution of the chapter authors. These beloved colleagues shared their time and professional expertise by writing the chapters, and I am incredibly indebted to them: Abdallah Rothman, Dr. Layla Asamarai, Farah Lodi, Dr. Afshana Haque, Dr. Ibrahim Rüschoff, Paul M. Kaplick, Dr. Rabia Malik, Hooman Keshavarzi, Dr. Fahad Khan, Dr. Fyeqa Sheikh, and Dr. Sayyed Mohsen Fatemi. Each of them also reviewed the Introduction that I wrote and provided important feedback. These are the people on the front lines helping to heal the hearts and minds of so many people in distress—such sacred work they are doing and they all have a special place in my heart!

I would also like to take a moment to say thank you to other beloved colleagues who have shared their work with me over the years. Although they do not have a chapter in this edited volume, many of them could have and all of them are doing incredibly important work: Dr. Nazila Isgandarova, Dr. Jalaledin Ebrahim, Karim Serageldin, Dr. Mahdi Qasqas, Dr. Sima Sweid, Mona Elgohail, Dr. Sameera Ahmed, Reem Suqi, Dr. Venus Mahmoodi, Khalida Haque, Najwa Awad, Dr. Ahmed Hassan, Dr. Sara Betteridge, Dr. Othman Mohammed, Dr. Rania Awaad, Madeeha Channah, Dr. Mona Amer, Dr. Khalid Elzamzamy, Dr. Khashayar Farhadi Langroudi, Ibrahim Jarrod Long, Seyma Saritoprak, and Dr. Marwa Assar. These people also have a special place in my heart!

Many thanks are also in order to the individuals who reviewed the Introduction in an extremely short period of time. Their feedback was incredibly valuable, and I have enormous admiration for them and am deeply indebted to these individuals. Indeed, they are all leaders in their fields, and I'm so honored they shared their expertise: Dr. Amber Haque, Dr. Malik Badri, Dr. P. Scott Richards, Dr. Timothy Sisemore, Dr. Hamada Hamid, Virginia Gray Henry, and Nasima Khanom—may you be rewarded beyond measure for your efforts.

I'd also like to acknowledge and thank the University of Iowa and specifically the departments in which I have a faculty appointment—Religious Studies and International Studies—as well as the faculty there who have enthusiastically supported my work on Islamic Psychology. Dr. Diana Fritz Cates, DEO of the Department of Religious Studies; Dr. Morten Schlutter, incoming DEO; my colleagues Dr. Ahmed Souaiaia and Dr. Kristy Nabhan-Warren; and the incredible support staff—Maureen Walterhouse and Robin Burns. Many thanks also go to the director and associate director of International Studies, Dr. Emily Wentzell and Dr. Karmen Berger, respectively.

Given that this is a book on psychotherapy and I speak in the Preface about my personal experience with it, and given that psychotherapists often go unnamed and publicly unthanked—indeed in order to maintain confidentiality, therapists tell their clients that if they see them in public they will not acknowledge them unless the client does so first—I would like to publicly acknowledge and thank my own therapists who have also been great teachers and mentors to me: Cyntha Gonzalez, an absolute beloved soul and who started it all for me many years ago in Dubai, as well as other healers at that time with whom I did alternative work, particularly Andrea Anstiss and Helen Wade. I would also like to thank Dr. Volker Thomas for recently helping us through a pretty stressful period of time—absolutely no shame in having needed any of your help!

Last, but certainly not least, I owe endless thanks and have immense gratitude to my very large and wonderful family. To my husband, Dr. Ahmed Alkaram, who is amazing, loving, intelligent, humble, and not to mention an extremely talented surgeon—no better husband exists on the face of the earth! So far we have spent ten fantastic years together, and during that time he has provided our entire family with such a wonderful life. His generosity has also afforded me the luxury of being able to work when I want and to choose to do only the projects that I absolutely love—such an incredible gift. To our wonderful daughter Lina, who is only seven, but is the most precious thing on the face of the planet—I could not have asked for a more special child. To my dear step-children—Farooq, twenty-one; Hajer, twenty; and Yaser, nineteen—I am so grateful that Lina has siblings who absolutely adore her and whom she loves back even more. Indeed their invaluable help in caring for her does not go unnoticed or unappreciated. To my mother-in-law, Bushra, who lives with us, she helps keep our life going, whether it's cooking, watching Lina or the other kids (when they were younger), and just being a stable presence in the house. My gratitude is immense.

And to my family members who do not live in my immediate household but who contribute enormously to my life. My parents, Nathan York and Glenda Duell; my step-parents, Cheryl York and Kent Duell; my siblings, Jarrod York, Luke Duell, and Karl Duell, and their spouses and children; my step-siblings, Mark Burke, Steven MacJarrett (who is no longer with us), Tiffany MacJarrett, Reigan Quintal, and Jude Lehman, and their spouses and children. I also want to acknowledge my grandparents who are, except one, still alive and in amazing health: my paternal grandmother Lois York, ninety-three (my paternal grandfather,

Herbert York, died before I was born); my maternal grandfather, Maynard Baker, eighty-eight; and my maternal grandmother, Ruth Wadsworth, eighty-one. All of these people have impacted the person I am today and all of them have a very special place in my heart. I want to publicly acknowledge them all.

Preface

MENTAL HEALTH and psychological treatment are highly stigmatized in the Muslim community. Although there are many reasons for this, two major ones stand out and served as guideposts as we
put together this book. First is the idea that Western psychotherapy is
antithetical to Islam. Although this might have been true historically,
particularly in the mid-twentieth century, and it still is today with some
approaches, in the past twenty years the tide has changed significantly,
with Muslim clinicians being at the forefront of developing theoretical
models and interventions that *do* take into account an Islamic worldview,
and in some cases are based on it. The chapters in this book are evidence
of how this is being done and what some of this work looks like. Second,
is the pervasive yet dangerous idea that praying and increasing one's
faith is all that a Muslim needs to do to deal with psychological distress.
Although the evidence suggests that prayer and other spiritual resources
can be an incredible source of comfort during difficult times, religion
and spirituality are not a cure-all. Failure to properly understand the
complex and nuanced relationship between religion, spirituality, and
mental health causes confusion and perpetuates stigma. Given this context of stigma combined with the growing amount of exceptional work
being done in the field of Islamically integrated psychotherapy, we felt
it an opportune time to bring this work to the public.

We had three primary audiences in mind when putting together this
edited volume. First and foremost is the everyday Muslim. Indeed, our
intention was to shine a light on the therapeutic encounter in which
Western psychotherapy and Islam engage with each other. We hope
that increased knowledge in this regard will decrease stigma. Second,

we wrote the material with other Muslim clinicians in mind. We also hope that sharing some of the ways colleagues are practicing Islamically integrated psychotherapy will prove useful to them in their own practice. Finally, the work presented in this book should be beneficial to non-Muslim clinicians who want to increase their knowledge about ways they could tailor services for their Muslim clients. In that regard, the book's content will speak to readers differently, depending on the angle from which they approach it.

It is important to me that readers know that I have done my best to do this project as comprehensively as I possibly could. My aim was to provide a global perspective of the topic, primarily positioned within the modern context of psychology and psychotherapy, and to bring unity to this growing field. However, like all books on any given topic, there are a variety of ways it can be done as well as limitations to its scope. In terms of limitations, please consider the following. First, although the chapter authors are located in various countries throughout the world, I fully acknowledge that at least the Introduction is still more Western-oriented (particularly American). Covering all regions of the globe equally, especially where English is not the language of research or publication, is a huge undertaking. Moreover, the situation of mental health and psychological care in Muslim-majority countries is complex and of a different nature than it is in the West, and it is simply too vast of a topic; indeed that could be a whole other book. Additionally, since it is from a contemporary perspective, I did not provide an extensive historical overview of psychology or psychotherapy in the ancient Muslim world, or of "psychotherapy" in the Islamic tradition. These are important yet also vast areas of scholarship that I have pointed to in the Introduction, and so have the authors in their individual chapters, but I did not want to replicate what has been done so well already in the literature or digress from the main theme. Despite these limitations, I hope the way this edited volume has been put together does satisfactory justice to the subject matter at hand.

I would also like to take a moment to share a few personal words from my heart that relate to the topic of this book. My first encounter with psychotherapy was as a client. I was in my twenties and living in Dubai (I'm in my forties now). My therapist, an American woman, definitely practiced spiritually integrated psychotherapy (although she called it transpersonal counseling), and it had such a profound impact on me that it literally changed the trajectory of my life. Personally, the insight I gained transformed me. I was able to make sense of my life in light of my childhood experiences and connect those dots to what was happening to me as an adult; it was like a light switched on. Professionally, I decided to enroll in a doctorate program and actually become a psychologist because I wanted to bring all that I had learned to the world, although at that time I did not envision it would be specifically within the context of Islam.

I realize that not everyone will have such a positive and transformational experience with psychotherapy, but I still believe that it has the potential of being immensely helpful to anyone who honestly gives it a chance and truly wants to change, even though it is often painful. Of course that doesn't mean that it's a cure-all or easy. However, if one truly has a sincere intention to deal with and heal from whatever is causing distress or dysfunction, I firmly believe that God will open doors to facilitate that process. For me, that process began with spiritually integrated psychotherapy. I have never personally had much stigma associated with it and have openly and often shared my experience, but I realize that is not the case for everyone. Indeed, as previously discussed, enormous shame surrounds psychological treatment. In my own personal attempt to model a positive help-seeking attitude and to destigmatize it, I am intentionally using this public platform to put into readers' minds the image of a specific person (me) who has gone to and benefited from psychotherapy. I hope this will encourage and inspire others to seek it when needed, even if they are ashamed to do so at first. It may be that you dislike a thing that is good for you (Quran 2:216).

My work is very much facilitated by my regular and supererogatory spiritual practices. I am not in a position to evaluate its quality, but I am extremely honored and humbled to have led this project through to completion and to share it with the public. I have given it my absolute best.

May peace and blessings be upon you.

Carrie York Al-Karam, PhD
March 2018
Iowa City, Iowa
United States of America

Islamically Integrated Psychotherapy

Introduction

ISLAMICALLY INTEGRATED PSYCHOTHERAPY (IIP) is a modern approach or orientation to psychotherapy that integrates Islamic teachings, principles, philosophies, and/or interventions with Western therapeutic approaches. IIP is also sometimes referred to as Islamic counseling or Islamic psychotherapy, although there is scholarly debate about the difference between these terms (for example, what constitutes "Islamic," the difference between counseling and psychotherapy, as well as how those terms are understood from within the Islamic tradition). Of course, psychotherapy is not new within an Islamic context. Indeed, some of the early "doctors of the self/soul" were Muslims, and some of their historical contributions to psychology and mental health have been documented (for example, see publications in the psychological literature by Amber Haque, Nazila Isgandarova, Malik Badri, and Rania Awaad). Moreover, many have argued that the domain of Islamic spirituality (*tasawwuf*/Sufism/*tazkiyat al-nafs* [purification of the self/soul]) is essentially Islam's version of psychotherapy.

There are an endless number of ways to practice IIP. First of all, quite a number of psychotherapeutic approaches exist. The American Psychological Association (APA) organizes them into five broad categories: psychoanalysis and psychodynamic therapies, behavior therapy, cognitive therapy, humanistic therapy, and integrative or holistic therapy (APA, 2018). Second, there are so many religious teachings, principles, philosophies, and/or interventions relevant to psychotherapy and issues with which clients present that the number of permutations that could result as a combination of the two domains is nearly endless. Indeed, the individual chapters in this edited volume provide insight into the variety of Islamically integrated approaches. Before getting into the specifics of what those approaches look like, though, the purpose of this introductory chapter is to familiarize the reader with some of the scholarly domains in which IIP could be situated. The domains discussed here include the Psychology of Religion and Spirituality, Multicultural Psychology and Counseling, Transpersonal Psychology, Muslim Mental Health, and Islamic Psychology. Being acquainted with this broader landscape should provide some context for the emergence of Islamically integrated psychotherapy. Such an overview should also serve as an important resource on this topic in general. Following the delineation of those domains, an overview of the individual chapters is then provided. Finally and in closing, recommendations for ways forward within the field of IIP are offered.

Context

PSYCHOLOGY OF RELIGION AND SPIRITUALITY

It is still often believed that Western psychology does not accommodate religion; it is perceived to be a secular science having antireligion sympathies or that at least takes a neutral stance. Indeed, early figures such as Freud said religion was a pathology that needed to be cured. Despite a somewhat antagonistic history, religion and spirituality have still always had some sort of a presence in Western psychology. Early founders such as William James and others were deeply interested in issues of religion and spiritually (for example, see *Varieties of Religious Experience*, 1902), and in some cases were themselves religious people. In the last forty years, there has been a growing and now considerable presence of scholarship in the domain referred to as the Psychology of Religion and Spirituality (PRS), but unless one is familiar with or engaged in this subfield, it sometimes goes unaccounted for in the mainstream discourse and literature. Division 36 of the APA, the Society for the Psychology of Religion and Spirituality, was formally established in 1976, although it started off in 1946 as the American Catholic Psychological Association (see Reuder, 1999). The International Association for the Psychology of Religion was founded even earlier in the twentieth century in Europe. By now, there are numerous important PRS textbooks and handbooks, as well as peer-reviewed journals dedicated to the topic (see the *Journal for the Psychology of Religion and Spirituality*, the *International Journal for the Psychology of Religion*, *Spirituality in Clinical Practice*, the *Journal of Religion and Health*, and the *Journal of Mental Health, Religion & Culture*).

As a subfield of psychology, PRS scholars study everything from religious conversion, spiritual struggles, prayer, spirituality and health, and complementary and alternative therapies to nonbelief and atheism. There is even a whole body of psychological literature that discusses the operationalizing of religion, spirituality, and other faith terms (see Harris et al., 2018, for a thirty-year definitional content analysis of such terms). As per its relevance to IIP, PRS houses a field of scholarship known as "integration," which is essentially the combination (or integration) of psychology and theology. Within an applied context it is known as spiritually integrated psychotherapy (SIP), with IIP being SIP within an Islamic context.

A robust number of publications—including landmark books, articles, as well as the establishment of peer-reviewed journals on the topic of SIP—have skyrocketed over the past twenty years. By far, the bulk of this work has been done mostly in the West and in the area of Christian counseling and psychotherapy, but noteworthy contributions can also been seen in the domains of other traditions, especially in Buddhism. Landmark books specifically on the topic of integrating religion and spirituality into psychotherapy and that are of significant importance to this edited volume are *Handbook of Psychotherapy and Religious Diversity* (Richards & Bergin, 2000, 2014), *A Spiritual Strategy for Counseling and Psychotherapy* (Richards & Bergin, 2005), *Spiritually Oriented Psychotherapy* (Sperry & Shafranske, 2004), and *Spiritually Integrated Psychotherapy: Understanding and Addressing the Sacred* (Pargament, 2007), to name a few, not to mention thousands of articles in the scientific literature on the topic. A synthesis of publications and a delineation of accomplishments in this field was recently undertaken by Richards, Sanders, Lea, McBride, and Allen (2015). Their findings highlight those accomplishments, some of which include:

- » Longstanding historical and philosophical biases against religion and spirituality were confronted (Bergin, 1980; Griffin, 2000; Jones, 1994; Slife & Williams, 1995).

▸ Alternative philosophical and theological perspectives that are more open to spirituality have been articulated (Bergin, 1980; Griffin, 2000; Miller, 2012; Richards & Bergin, 2005; Slife, 2004).

▸ Hundreds of research studies have demonstrated the therapeutic potential of religious lifestyles and personal spirituality (e.g., Koenig, McCullough, & Larson, 2001).

▸ Theoretical and clinical literature is now widely available that provides insight into how practitioners can ethically and effectively integrate spiritual perspectives and interventions into health care treatment. Spiritually oriented psychotherapy approaches grounded in the healing practices of both Western and Eastern spiritual traditions have been described (Pargament, 2007; Richards & Bergin, 2005; Sperry & Shafranske, 2005).

▸ Many spiritual approaches have been integrated with mainstream secular theories, including Jungian, transpersonal, psychodynamic, cognitive-behavioral, and rational-emotive therapy, and interpersonal, humanistic, and multicultural approaches (Richards & Bergin, 2004; Sperry & Shafranske, 2005).

▸ Many health care practitioners have embraced the importance of religion and spirituality in treatment and incorporate spiritually oriented approaches into their clinical work (Jackson, 2014; Post, Cornish, Wade, & Tucker, 2013; Raphel, 2001; Richards & Potts, 1995; Shafranske, 2000; Wade, Worthington, & Vogel, 2007). Most practitioners integrate spiritual approaches in treatment tailoring them with mainstream secular approaches to psychotherapy (Richards & Bergin, 2004, 2005).

▸ Psychotherapy outcome studies provide evidence that spiritually oriented treatment approaches are effective (Anderson et al., 2015; Hook et al., 2010; McCullough, 1999; Smith, Bartz, & Richards, 2007; Worthington, Hook, Davis, & McDaniel, 2011; Worthington, Kurusu, McCollough, & Sanders, 1996; Worthington & Sandage, 2001).

In response to these achievements, a groundbreaking initiative called

Bridges Consortium was established (www.bridgesconsortium.com) whose mission and vision are to build bridges between spiritual and secular approaches to psychotherapy and to help bridge the research-practice gap in the health care profession (Richards et al., 2015). Also from this initiative emerged one of the biggest studies to date that seeks to explore processes and outcomes of spiritually integrated psychotherapy from a variety of religious traditions and is now being undertaken (2017–2021) and partially funded with a $3.57 million grant from the John Templeton Foundation; its title is *Bringing Spiritually Integrated Psychotherapy into the Healthcare Mainstream*. Results from this big-data study will start to come in as early as 2018. (See the Keshavarzi and Khan chapter in this book for details of the sole Islamic modality being investigated in this twenty-two-project study. Coinvestigators are Fahad Khan and Hooman Keshavarzi, Carrie York Al-Karam, and Mawlana Bilal Ali Ansari, representing the Khalil Center, the Al-Karam Lab for Islamic Psychology, and Darul Qasim, respectively.)

Multicultural Psychology and Counseling

Multicultural psychology and counseling, a field that bridges a variety of disciplines from which psychotherapists come, including psychology and social work, grew out of a recognition that the ethnic, racial, and/or cultural background of an individual must be taken into account in the psychotherapeutic encounter, with religion and spirituality being a component of "culture." The Indigenous Psychology movement (Enriquez, 1990; Allwood & Berry, 2006; Kim, Yang, & Hwang, 2006) has also emerged in connection with this domain and posits that *all* psychology is indigenous (Marcella, 2013), including Western psychology. Marcella (2013) notes:

> While the term "indigenous" is often used to refer to "native" people and cultures, post-modern ideological and socio-political uses of the term have resulted in a growing opinion among psychologists that all psychologies are "indigenous" to the cultures in which they arise and are sustained. This posi-

tion challenges the current dominance and privileged stance of Western (i.e., Eurocentric/North American) psychology as a universal set of assumptions, methods and applications.

From a multicultural or indigenous perspective, in order to provide appropriate psychological care, therapeutic models must emerge from within the indigenous system(s) in which any given client is positioned because people and the cultures from which they come cannot be disconnected from basic psychological processes, as these are culturally bound (indigenization from within), or therapeutic models from divergent cultures need to be fitted to the particular cultural context of the client (indigenization from without). Examples of competencies that a multicultural therapist should possess are numerous, some of which include knowledge about the client's cultural group's history; family structures, gender roles, and dynamics; response to illness; "culture-specific" disorders; indigenous healing methods and explanatory models of illness; and communication patterns and styles, to name a few. Although religious psychologies can transcend some of the markers typically associated with indigenous psychologies such as culture, language, ethnicity, and geographical location, some researchers are now arguing that religious psychologies, such as Islamic psychology, are indigenous (see Haque & Masuan, 2002; Skinner, 2015; Ward, 2017).

Transpersonal Psychology

Including spiritual practices and therapies into the therapeutic setting is the cornerstone of transpersonal psychotherapy (TP). Transpersonal psychologists are interested in the experiences and practices of the world's great religious traditions, as well as altered states of consciousness and spiritual issues in mental health (Lukoff, 2000, p. 81). From a transpersonal perspective, psychotherapy is about helping and supporting the individual to connect with and experience his or her whole self, including the relationship to the Divine (Boorstein, 2000; Firman & Gila, 2002). In terms of TP's relevance specifically within an Islamic context, not only has Islam-related psychological scholarship been done within its domain (for example, see York, 2011; Lazarus, 1985), Robert Frager, one of TP's most influential figures and founder of Sofia University (formerly the Institute of Transpersonal Psychology), is a Muslim and Sufi sheikh who has written extensively on Sufism and the wisdom of Islam within a psycho-spiritual context.

Muslim Mental Health

Islamically integrated psychotherapy has also emerged from an area known as Muslim Mental Health (MMH). MMH's main focus has been to understand the mental health needs of Muslims, primarily living in the West and in a post–September 11, 2001, world, and to have a collective voice in addressing those needs (Basit & Hamid, 2006). Literature emerging from this domain shows that Muslims tend to be more reluctant in seeking mental health treatment for their psychological distress relative to other groups (Sheikh & Furnham, 2000; Pilkington, Msetfi, & Watson, 2012); religious, spiritual, and cultural sensitivities are concerns that Muslims have about therapy, which in turn adversely impact their help-seeking behaviors (Inayat, 2007; Aloud & Rathur, 2009; Haque & Mohamed, 2009) and Muslims often avoid seeking psychotherapy services if the therapist does not provide it within a religious or spiritual context (Amri & Bemak, 2013; Killawi et al., 2014). Moreover, even mental health professions such as psychology, psychiatry, and social work are stigmatized, particularly in Muslim-majority countries, with many Muslims being discouraged by their families from taking up careers in these domains.

Early markers of the MMH field began, at least in the United States, with the establishment of the Institute of Muslim Mental Health (IMMH) in 2006; its peer-reviewed scientific journal founded the same year, the *Journal of Muslim Mental Health*; and an annual conference that began in 2008. During this annual conference, experts present research and discuss pressing Muslim mental health concerns ranging from Islamophobia, war and forced migration, substance abuse, domestic violence, radicalization, coping and help-seeking behaviors, as well as mental health first-aid training for Imams, chaplains, and other religious leaders as they are, at times, first responders for Muslims dealing with mental health issues. Indeed, one could argue that the theoretical underpinnings of Muslim chaplaincy and IIP, such as how mental/spiritual health, illness, and healing are conceptualized, are effectively the same, although the scope of practice of chaplains and psychotherapists differ in a modern Western context. The professionalization of Muslim chaplaincy, as seen in the establishment of degree programs at Hartford Seminary and Bayan Claremont to name two institutions, as well as the Association of Muslim Chaplains, is of significant importance within the context of the MMH landscape.

Landmark texts that further consolidated the MMH movement were *Counseling and Psychotherapy with Arabs and Muslims* (Dwairy, 2006), *Counseling Muslims: Handbook of Mental Health Issues and Interventions* (Ahmed & Amer, 2012), *Islamic Counseling: An Introduction to Theory and Practice* (Rassool, 2016), and *Family Therapy with Muslims* (Daneshpour, 2016). Other noteworthy developments in MMH can be seen in the establishment of a number of institutions, including the Family and Youth Institute (2006), Naseeha—Muslim Youth Helpline (2006), Mental Health 4 Muslims (2009), Khalil Center (2010), Stones to Bridges (2010), the Muslim Wellness Foundation (2012), the Muslims and Mental Health Lab at Stanford University (2014), the American Muslim Health Professionals Mental Health section, as well as a whole host of private psychotherapy practices too numerous to list here that are both owned by and cater to Muslims.

Parallel developments have been happening in Europe during the past twenty-five years or so, especially the United Kingdom. Examples include the Institute of Islamic Counseling and Wellbeing in London (1996), the Ihsaan Islamic Psychological Therapy Service (2014) in Bradford, Al-Inayat, and the Lateef Project. Additionally, professional networks have been formed, such as the Muslim Counsellor and Psychotherapist Network (MCAPN). In Germany, the Islamic Association of Social and Educational Professions was established (1989) as was its Islam and Psychology research group (2015).

In terms of Muslim-majority countries, mental health and psychological services are less developed than they are in the West, although this situation can vary greatly depending on the particular country or region in question. In general, though, when services or degree and training programs are available, they are often imported part and parcel from the West (which perpetuates stigmatization), although this is definitely starting to change. For example, see the chapter in this book by Layla Asamarai on IIP in the United Arab Emirates as well as Farah Lodi's chapter on the HEART method of counseling. Another example is a forthcoming psychology textbook that was designed specifically for use in the Arab Gulf (*An Introduction to Psychology for the Arabian Gulf*, Lambert & Pasha-Zaidi, 2018) that has sections on mental health from an Islamic perspective as well as a full chapter on Islamic psychology.

What is presented here is not an exhaustive review of all institutions, individuals, or developments in the global field of MMH. At the time of this writing, a scan of the Internet and social media on MMH reveals an explosion of activity in this domain globally—conferences, private clinics, blogs, vlogs, YouTube talks, and self-help courses, as well as an increase in the number of mental health professionals (psychologists, psychiatrists, social workers, etc.) who are Muslims, and in some cases who are also trained in the Islamic sciences. That said, hopefully what has been presented here provides enough context to have a better idea about an important domain from which IIP has emerged.

Islamic Psychology

Another area in which IIP can be situated is the field of Islamic Psychology (IP). There continues to be scholarly debate as to what IP is, how it is defined, and the parameters of the discipline (see York Al-Karam, 2017). For example, some consider IP to be synonymous with the work of early Muslim scholars such as al-Ghazali, al-Balkhi, al-Razi, and others. Indeed, numerous articles in the contemporary psychological literature have synthesized the works of these early "doctors of the self/ soul" (Badri, 2014; Haque, 2004; Awaad & Ali, 2015, 2016; Isgandarova, 2018) as well as some of the "psychotherapies" they practiced (for example, see Badri, 2014; Isgandarova, 2018). One could argue that the whole area of Islamic spirituality (Sufism / *tasawwuf, tazkiyat al-nafs*, etc.) is actually Islam's version of what we today call psychotherapy and some consider *that* to be IP.

Regardless of how it might be defined or conceptualized, IP's emergence in the modern context is usually associated with the Islamization of Knowledge (IOK) movement (al-Attas, 1993; al-Faruqi, 1982) and later the Indigenous Psychology movement previously discussed. Although there are different ways the IOK movement has been conceptualized, Islamization essentially attempts to reconcile Islam and modernity without compromising Islamic ethical and intellectual principles. The philosophy aims to bring change to the Muslim thought process and encourages Muslims to evaluate and practice knowledge from an Islamic epistemological perspective (Haque, 2018). As it relates specifically to psychology, Malik Badri (b. 1932), a British-educated Sudanese, was one of the first and perhaps most influential Muslim psychologists in modern times to call for the Islamization of psychology in his now classic publication, *The Dilemma of a Muslim Psychologist* (1979). According to Badri (2009), not all of psychology needs to be Islamized, particularly the parts of the discipline related to biology, chemistry (such as hormones, neurotransmitters, etc.), anatomy (e.g., of the brain), or of sensorial processes such as perception. Rather, it is the areas of psychology that deal with theories of personality, abnormal psychology, humanistic psychology (that relies on existential philosophy), and most of the schools of psychotherapy (Badri, 2009, p. 9) that need to be Islamized so that a science based on an Islamic understanding of the self, including what constitutes pathology and healing, can emerge. A number of noteworthy publications in the psychological literature speak to this point, particularly on the nature and structure of the self/personality from an Islamic perspective (for example, see Haque & Mohamed, 2009; Abu-Raiya, 2012, 2014; Keshavarzi and Haque, 2013; Haque and Keshavarzi, 2012). As for the Islamization of psychotherapy, certainly the chapters in this book demonstrate some of the ways this is currently happening.

In terms of global institutional markers of an emerging IP discipline, much work has been coming out of the International Islamic University Malaysia (IIUM), which was founded in 1983 as a project of the IOK movement. In fact, Badri was a professor in the Psychology Department there for many years. Badri also went on to found the International Association of Muslim Psychologists (1997), which is still quite active in Malaysia. IP courses are also now being offered at Cambridge Muslim College in the United Kingdom (taught by Rasjid Skinner) and the University of Iowa in the United States (taught by Carrie York Al-Karam), as well as an IP degree program at Aligargh Muslim University in India (headed by Akbar Husain). Jamia Millia Islamia houses the Indian Council of Islamic Perspective in Psychology (founded in 2015) and collaborates with Aligarh Muslim University as well as the Centre for Research and Study in Hyderabad, India. Forthcoming degree programs in IP are expected at Istanbul Zaim University in Turkey, and Neelain University in Sudan, both of which are connected to the work of Professor Badri and his establishing in 2017 the International Association of Islamic Psychology (IAIP). One of the aims of IAIP is to provide accreditation to IP programs throughout the world in order to establish standards of practice, although the establishment of this organization will not be formally announced until October 2018 in Turkey. The *Journal of Islamic Psychology* and an annual Islamic psychology conference are also housed in IAIP. Additionally, the Islamic Psychology Professional Association was established in 2015 in the United Kingdom, and its aim is to develop Islamic approaches to psychology for psychotherapy and allied health and social care fields. Indeed, like its MMH counterpart, IP is an emerging domain in which much scholarly interest continues to develop. What is presented here is by no means a comprehensive overview, and indeed the landscape is changing constantly.

The Chapters

Each chapter in this volume was written by a Muslim licensed clinician who regularly provides psychotherapy to Muslim clients. In an attempt to destigmatize and demystify the process, they have provided a bird's-eye view of how they incorporate religion and spirituality into their psychotherapeutic service delivery. Authors were asked to address the following points in their chapters:

- ▸ What their primary therapeutic orientations(s) are (CBT, psychoanalysis, humanistic, family/couples, etc.)
- ▸ Whether these therapeutic orientations are "Islam friendly" or if they have concepts/philosophies that are at odds with certain Islamic beliefs and to discuss congruence and/or dissonance
- ▸ What Islamic teachings, principles, or interventions they use in therapy and how they go about it
- ▸ If their approach is a "bottom-up" or indigenous approach (importing Western strategies/philosophies into an otherwise inherently Islamic approach) or a "top-down" or exogenous approach (bringing Islam into Western psychotherapy)
- ▸ What guides them in their practice of integration
- ▸ How they deal with differences in theological interpretation
- ▸ What challenges they face practicing spiritually integrated psychotherapy
- ▸ Whether they use any measurements to assess treatment outcomes, and if so, which ones

They were also asked to provide vignettes or case studies that exemplify the work and to make recommendations for ways forward.

In chapter 1, "An Islamic Theoretical Orientation to Psychotherapy," Abdallah Rothman begins by distinguishing between MMH and IP and asserts the existence of and need for a uniquely Islamic paradigm of human psychology. He goes on to describe how Islam can be viewed as a system for psychological well-being or a "science of the soul" and how he operates from within an Islamic theoretical orientation to psychology. He concludes by giving examples from his clinical practice of how he works with his clients by employing uniquely Islamic therapeutic interventions derived from the Islamic tradition.

In chapter 2, "Utilization of Islamic Principles in Marital Counseling," Layla Asamarai, a clinical psychologist who practiced for over eight years in Dubai, United Arab Emirites, shares a number of deidentified vignettes from her clinical work with couples. As she describes her clients' dilemmas, she brings the reader on board in appreciating the dilemma and the Islamically informed approach that she utilized in working with the given clients.

In chapter 3, "The HEART Method: Healthy Emotions Anchored in RasoolAllah's Teachings: Cognitive Therapy Using Prophet Mohammed as a Psycho-Spiritual Exemplar," Farah Lodi offers an analysis of how Prophet Mohammed remained consistently hopeful and positive even during the most difficult times of his life. She has created a counseling method consisting of six key teachings exemplified by the Prophet in his lifetime. She describes how he practiced each strategy, cites how it is discussed in the Quran, and links these prophetic examples to evidence-based research in modern psychological literature. Finally she suggests practical ways to help clients embrace these teachings.

In chapter 4, "Conducting Spiritually Integrated Family Therapy with Muslim Clients Utilizing a Culturally Responsive Paradigm," Afshana Haque describes the use of Islamically integrated family therapy through a culturally responsive lens. After emphasizing the importance of considering many Muslims' double-minority status, she provides various clinical case examples to illustrate the application of this model with the use of the collaborative language systems paradigm. Finally, she highlights challenges she experiences when using this model and also suggests indications for including spirituality in a therapy session.

In chapter 5, "Integrating Islamic Spirituality into Psychodynamic Therapy with Muslim Patients," Ibrahim Rüsschoff and Paul Kaplick describe how Islamic spiritual elements can be integrated into psychodynamic therapy and psychoanalytical object relations theory in particular, to the benefit of Muslim patients. Case studies illustrate why a Muslim practitioner is pivotal in addressing the specific psycho-spiritual needs of Muslim patients, how Allah's ninety-nine names can be employed in the biographical work with Muslim patients, that psychodynamic therapy is appropriate to treat a number of case presentations including the panic disorder of an Imam, and ways in which psychotherapists can approach Muslim patients who explain clinical symptomatology with black magic and *jinn*. The chapter suggests that a top-down approach, which integrates Islamic spiritual elements into psychodynamic therapy, is upholding both Islamic and professional psychotherapeutic work standards. Thereby, the authors counteract a general trend in the Islamic psychological literature that demonizes psychoanalysis and psychodynamic therapy and erroneously renders its application in the psychotherapy of Muslim patients unfitting.

In chapter 6, "Family Therapy and the Use of Quranic Stories," Rabia Malik begins by describing what drew her to systemic therapy and why she thinks theoretically systemic theory has the capacity to include religious and spiritual contexts in understanding the psychological needs of Muslim clients. She goes on to illustrate how she has integrated the use of Quranic stories with the Coordinated Management of Meaning (CMM) model to explore and challenge how religious beliefs or "stories told" are interwoven into people's relationships and vice versa, and how our experiences of "stories lived" can make us rethink religious beliefs. She concludes that in order to integrate Islamic beliefs with therapeutic practices, a more critical approach toward both needs to be taken, challenging dominant ethnocentric assumptions inherent in most therapeutic approaches, as well as creating an exploratory space that may be challenging for dominant authoritarian interpretations of Islam.

Hooman Keshavarzi and Fahad Khan in chapter 7, "Outlining a Case Example of Islamically Integrated Psychotherapy," describe a case illustration of what they have come to term traditional Islamically integrated psychotherapy (TIIP). This modality is based upon a classical Islamic theoretical framework that is integrative of modern behavioral science. This framework outlines an Islamic epistemological and ontological schema for the integration of modern psychological strategies toward achieving psycho-spiritual health. They demonstrate the practical usage of this framework across sessions in the treatment of a patient with social anxiety. Interventions are either inherently Islamically indigenous or they are adaptations of modern psychological techniques that are congruent with the Islamic underpinnings and objectives of the model.

In chapter 8, "Marrying Islamic Principles with Western Psychotherapy for Children and Adolescents: Successes and Challenges," Fyeqa Sheikh describes various challenges in working with Muslim children and adolescents as well as their families. Through the use of case examples, she delineates how she has overcome these challenges in psychotherapy and her unique process of integrating Islamic principles into

Western, cognitive behavioral therapy (CBT)-oriented strategies. She further discusses difficulties with creating a framework for Islamic psychotherapy, while also offering recommendations for unifying the discipline.

In the final chapter, "Integrating *Duaa* of *Arafa* and Other Shiite Teachings into Psychotherapy," Sayyed Mohsen Fatemi, presenting the sole chapter from a Shiite perspective, discusses the use of various Islamic teachings in psychotherapy and their implications for well-being. Specifically, he focuses on the *duaa* of *Arafa* and explicates its facilitating function in helping the client to renew his or her perspective when dealing with stressful situations, depression, and anxiety.

Moving Forward

Muslims should no longer cling to mental health stigma. The Islamic tradition urges people to seek healing, and the chapters in this book show that psychotherapeutic services that are based on an Islamic worldview are available now and this is what some of them look like. Moreover, given the current multicultural milieu that exists generally in the mental health domain, it could be argued that even non-Muslim therapists are more capable than ever of providing adequate therapy to Muslims. Of course, that doesn't mean we've "arrived" and no further work is needed, but it does provide an opportunity to reflect on what has been accomplished and where further work is required.

In terms of recommendations for next steps, first and foremost is to continue to educate the Muslim community to reduce stigma related to mental health. Efforts are well under way all across the globe, but more needs to be done. An important development in this regard, at least in North America, and that exemplifies what larger-scale MMH education could look like, is the recent establishment of a mental health task force by the Islamic Society of North America (ISNA), the largest Muslim organization in North America. For the first time in its fifty-five years, there will be an entire mental health program track at the annual convention in September 2018.

Second, more Muslims are needed in mental health

professions—psychology, psychiatry, social work, counseling, psychotherapy, psychiatric nursing. The field is vast. There is a great need for Muslims to be service providers, educators, and advocates, and to give a Muslim voice and perspective to the various fields in which they would serve.

Third, we need degree and training programs that produce these professionals, particularly programs that are housed in *accredited Muslim* institutions of higher education and that are based on the science of *Islamic* psychology. In the meantime, a variety of programs in psychology, psychotherapy, and counseling disciplines offer degrees in multicultural or "minority mental health," at least in the United States, and Muslims need to take advantage of these opportunities.

Fourth, Muslims must be active in and build the Muslim professional associations that already exist, some of which were previously mentioned. A large and growing number of individuals and institutions are dedicated to MMH, and it is important that these entities collaborate. Moreover, Muslims must also be actively involved in mainstream associations, including serving in leadership roles, especially when it comes to policy advocacy. Again, given the Zeitgeist of multiculturalism, the field of mental health wants to hear from and is calling for Muslim voices!

Fifth, we need research that explores these and other Islamically integrated psychotherapies. Such scholarship will likely have broad yet important implications for psychology and mental health as a whole.

Finally, and perhaps most importantly, I invite all Muslims to seriously reflect upon what is stated in the Quran, that "indeed, Allah will not change the condition of a people until they change what is in themselves" (13:11). When someone is in psychological or emotional pain; is depressed; is suffering from anxiety or post traumatic stress disorder (PTSD); has a substance abuse problem, marital or family conflict, or obsessive or suicidal thoughts; has experienced domestic violence or physical, verbal, or sexual abuse; or is just having difficulty dealing with the stressors of life, and this individual does not seek proper psychotherapeutic treatment, these unresolved psychological and emotional wounds become the veils that keep one disconnected from oneself, from others, and ultimately from God. Indeed, Prophet Mohammed said,

"Whosoever knows himself knows his Lord." Psychotherapy, whether it is integrated with spirituality or not, can be one way to obtain self-knowledge, thereby potentially being an avenue through which one can change one's condition and become closer to God. Moreover, it has been argued that the concept of psychotherapy is indigenous to the Islamic tradition and known as "purification of the self" (*tazkiyat al-nafs*). Given that God has said that those who purify themselves are successful (91:9), this should encourage all of us to consider psychotherapy, especially if underpinned by an Islamic worldview, as one way to achieve success, in this life and perhaps the next, *inshallah*.

References

Abu-Raiya, H. (2012). Towards a systematic Qura'nic theory of personality. *Mental Health, Religion & Culture, 15*(3), 217–233. doi:10.1080/13674676.2011.640622

Abu-Raiya, H. (2014). Western psychology and Muslim psychology in dialogue: Comparisons between a Qura'nic theory of personality and Freud's and Jung's ideas. *Journal of Religion & Health, 53*(2), 326–338. doi:10.1007/s10943-012-9630-9

Ahmed, S., & Amer, M. (2012). *Counseling Muslims: Handbook of mental health issues and interventions.* New York: Routledge.

Al-Attas, S. M. (1993). *Islam and secularism.* Kuala Lumpur, Malaysia: International Institute of Islamic Thought and Civilisation (ISTAC).

Al-Faruqi, I. R. (1982). *Islamization of knowledge: General principles and work plan.* Herndon, VA: International Institute of Islamic Thought.

Allwood, C. M., & Berry, J. W. (2006). Origins and development of indigenous psychologies: An international analysis. *International Journal of Psychology, 41*(4), 243–268. doi:10.1080/00207590544000013

Aloud, N., & Rathur, A. (2009). Factors affecting attitudes towards seeking and using formal mental health and psychological services among Arab Muslim populations. *Journal of Muslim Mental Health, 4*, 79–103.

American Psychological Association. (2018). *Different approaches to psychotherapy.* http://www.apa.org/topics/therapy/psychotherapy-approaches.aspx

Amri, S., & Bemak, F. (2013). Mental health help-seeking behaviors of Muslim immigrants in the United States: Overcoming social stigma and cultural mistrust. *Journal of Muslim Mental Health, 7*(1), 43–63.

Anderson, N., Heywood-Everett, S., Siddiqi, N., Wright, J., Meredith, J., & McMillan, D. (2015). Faith-adapted psychological therapies for depression and anxiety: Systematic review and meta-analysis. *Journal of Affective Disorders, 176,* 183–196. http://dx.doi.org/10.1016/j.jad.2015.01.019

Awaad, R., & Ali, S. (2015). Obsessional disorders in al-Balkhi's 9th-century treatise: Sustenance of the body and soul. *Journal of Affective Disorders, 180,* 185–189. doi:10.1016/j.jad.2015.03.003

Awaad, R., & Ali, S. (2016). A modern conceptualization of phobia in al-Balkhi's 9th-century treatise: Sustenance of the body and soul. *Journal of Anxiety Disorders, 37,* 89–93. doi:10.1016/j.janxdis.2015.11.003

Badri, M. (1979). *The Dilemma of Muslim Psychologists.* London: MWH London.

Badri, M. (1998). Al-Balkhi: A genius whose psychiatric contributions needed more than ten centuries to be appreciated. *Malaysian Journal of Psychiatry, 6*(2), 12–17.

Badri, M. (2009). *The Islamization of Psychology: Its "Why", Its "What", Its How" and Its "Who."* https://i-epistemology.net/vi/psychology/60-the-islamization-of-psychology-its-why-its-what-its-how-and-its-who.html

Badri, M. (2013). *Abū Zayd al-Balkhī's sustenance of the soul: The cognitive behavior therapy of a ninth-century physician.* London: International Institute of Islamic Thought.

Badri, M. (2014). *Emotional blasting therapy: A psychotherapeutic technique invented by early Muslim physicians.* Paper presented at Developing Synergies between Islam and Science & Technology for Mankind's Benefit, Kuala Lumpur, Malaysia.

Basit, A., & Hamid, H. (2006). Editors' introduction. *Journal of Muslim Mental Health, 1,* 1–3. doi: 10.1080/15564900600764911

Bergin, A. E. (1980). Psychotherapy and religious values. *Journal of Consulting and Clinical Psychology, 48,* 95–105. http://dx.doi.org/10.1037/0022-006X.48.1.95

Boorstein, S. (2000). Transpersonal psychotherapy. *American Journal of Psychotherapy, 54*(3), 408–424.

Daneshpour, M. (2016). *Family therapy with Muslims.* New York: Routledge.

Dwairy, M. (2006). Counseling and psychotherapy with Arabs and Muslims. New York: Teachers College Press.

Enriquez, V. G. (Ed.) (1990). *Indigenous psychology: A book of readings.* Quezon City, Philippines: Akademya ng Sikolohiyang Pilipino.

Firman, J., & Gila, A. (2002). *Psychosynthesis: A psychology of spirit.* Albany, NY: SUNY Press.

Griffin, D. R. (2000). *Religion and scientific naturalism: Overcoming the conflicts.* Albany, NY: SUNY Press.

Haque, A., & Masuan, K. A. (2002). Religious psychology in Malaysia. *International Journal for the Psychology of Religion, 12*(4), 277–289. doi:10.1207/s15327582ijpr1204_05

Haque, A. (2004). Psychology from Islamic perspective: Contributions of early Muslim scholars and challenges to contemporary Muslim psychologists. *Journal of Religion and Health, 43*(4), 357–377. doi:10.1007/s10943-004-4302-z

Haque, A. & Mohamed, Y. (2009). Psychology of personality: Islamic perspectives. Singapore: Cengage Learning Asia.

Haque, A., Khan, F., Keshavarzi, H., & Rothman, A. E. (2016). Integrating Islamic traditions in modern psychology: Research trends in last ten years. *Journal of Muslim Mental Health, 10*(1), 75-100.

Haque, A. & Keshavarzi, H. (2014). Integrating indigenous healing methods in therapy: Muslim beliefs and practices. *International Journal of Culture and Mental Health.* V7, 2014. P. 297-314.

Haque, A. (2018). Islamization of knowledge: The case of psychology. *Talk delivered to the Department of Islamic Studies – Aligarh Muslim University (India).* January 3rd, 2018.

Harris, K., Howell, D., & Spurgeon, D. (2018). Faith concepts in psychology: Three 30-year definitional content analyses. *Psychology of Religion and Spirituality,* Vol. 10(1), 1-29.

Hook, J. N., Worthington, E. L., Jr., Davis, D. E., Jennings, D. J., II, Gartner, A. L., & Hook, J. P. (2010). Empirically supported religious and spiritual therapies. *Journal of Clinical Psychology, 66,* 46–72.

Isgandarova, N. (2018). Multiple articles available from https://www.researchgate.net/profile/Nazila_Isgandarova

Inayat, Q. (2007). Islamophobia and the therapeutic dialogue: Some reflections. *Counselling Psychology Quarterly, 20*(3), 287–293.

Jackson, D. (2014). Reality therapy counselors using spiritual interventions in therapy. *International Journal of Choice Theory and Reality Therapy, 33,* 73–77.

James, W. (1902). *Varieties of religious experience: A study in human nature.* NY: Longmans, Green, & Co.

Johnson, E. L. (Ed.). (2010). *Psychology and Christianity. Five views.* Downers Grove, IL: InterVarsity Press.

Jones, S. L. (1994). A constructive relationship for religion with the science and profession of psychology: Perhaps the boldest model yet. *American Psychologist, 49,* 184–199. http://dx.doi.org/10.1037/0003-066X.49.3.184

Keshavarzi, H., & Haque, A. (2013). Outlining a psychotherapy model for enhancing Muslim mental health within an Islamic context. *International Journal for the Psychology of Religion, 23*(3), 230–249.

Killawi, A., Daneshpour, M., Elmi, A., Dadras, I., & Hamid, H. (2014). *Recommendations for promoting healthy marriages and preventing divorce in the American Muslim community.* http://www.ispu.org/pdfs/ISPU_Promoting_Healthy_

Marriages_and_Preventing_Divorce_in_the_American_Muslim_Community.pdf

Kim, U., & Berry, J. W. (1993). *Indigenous psychologies: Research and experience in cultural context.* Newbury Park, CA: Sage Publications.

Kim, U., Yang, K.-S., & Hwang, K.-K. (2006). Contributions to indigenous and cultural psychology: Understanding people in context. In U. Kim, K.-S. Yang, & K.-K. Hwang (Eds.), *Indigenous and cultural psychology: Understanding people in context* (pp. 3–25). New York: Springer.

Koenig, H. G., McCullough, M. E., & Larson, D. B. (2001). *Handbook of religion and health.* New York: Oxford University Press. http://dx.doi.org/10.1093/acprof:oso/9780195118667.001.0001

Lambert, L. & Pasha-Zaidi, N. (2018). *An Introduction to Psychology for the Arabian Gulf.* Cambridge Scholars Press.

Lazarus, I. (1985). *From Maslow to Muhammad: Maslow's description of self-actualization delineated in the life of Muhammad, pbuh.* Doctoral dissertation at the Institute of Transpersonal Psychology.

Lukoff, D. (2000). The importance of spirituality in mental health and mental illness. *Alternative Therapies in Health and Medicine, 6*(6), 80–88.

Marcella, A. (2013). *All psychologies are indigenous psychologies: Reflections on psychology in a global era.* http://www.apa.org/international/pi/2013/12/reflections.aspx

McCullough, M. E. (1999). Research on religion-accommodative counseling: Review and meta-analysis. *Journal of Counseling Psychology, 46,* 92–98. http://dx.doi.org/10.1037/0022-0167.46.1.92

Miller, L. (Ed.). (2012). *The Oxford handbook of psychology and spirituality.* New York: Oxford University Press. http://dx.doi.org/10.1093/oxfordhb/9780199729920.001.0001

Pargament, K. (2007). *Spiritually integrated psychotherapy: Understanding and addressing the sacred.* New York: Guilford Press.

Pilkington, A., Msetfia, RM., & Watson, R. (2012). Factors affecting intention to access psychological services amongst British Muslims of South Asian origin. Mental Health, Religion & Culture, 15(1), 1–22.

Post, B. C., Cornish, M. A., Wade, N. G., & Tucker, J. R. (2013). Religion and spirituality in group counseling: Beliefs and practices of university counseling center counselors. *Journal for Specialists in Group Work, 38,* 264–284. http://dx.doi.org/10.1080/01933922.2013.834401

Raphel, M. M. (2001). The status of the use of spiritual interventions in three professional mental health groups. *Dissertation Abstracts International, 62,* 779A.

Rassool, G. H. (2016). *Islamic counseling: An introduction to theory and practice.* New York: Routledge.

Reuder, M. (1999). A history of Division 36 (Psychology of Religion). In D. A. Dewsbury (Ed.), *Unification through division: Histories of the division of the American Psychological Association* (Vol. 4, pp. 91–108). Washington, DC: American Psychological Association, http://www.apadivisions.org/division-36/about/history.pdf

Richards, P. S., & Potts, R. W. (1995). Using spiritual interventions in psychotherapy: Practices, successes, failures, and ethical concerns of Mormon psychotherapists. *Professional Psychology: Re- search and Practice, 26,* 163–170. http://dx.doi.org/10.1037/0735-7028.26.2.163

Richards, P. S., & Bergin, A. (2000). *Handbook of psychotherapy and religious diversity.* Washington, DC: American Psychological Association.

Richards, P. S., & Bergin, A. E. (Eds.). (2004). *Casebook for a spiritual strategy in counseling and psychotherapy.* Washington, DC: American Psychological Association. http://dx.doi.org/10.1037/10652-000

Richards, P. S. & Bergin, A. (2005). *A spiritual strategy for counseling and psychotherapy.* Washington, DC: American Psychological Association.

Richards, P. S., & Bergin, A. (2014). *Handbook of psychotherapy and religious diversity* (2nd edition). Washington, DC: American Psychological Association.

Richards, P. S, Sanders, P. W., Lea, T., McBride, J. A., & Allen, G. E. K. (2015) Bringing spiritually oriented psychotherapies into the health care mainstream: *A Call for Worldwide Collaboration Spirituality in Clinical Practice, 2*(3), 169–179. doi:10.1037/scp0000082

Shafranske, E. P. (2000). Religious involvement and professional practices of psychiatrists and other mental health professionals. *Psychiatric Annals, 30,* 525–532. http://dx.doi.org/10.3928/0048-5713-20000801-07

Sheikh, S., & Furnham, A. (2000). A cross cultural study of mental health beliefs and attitudes towards seeking help. *Social Psychiatry and Psychiatric Epidemiology, 35,* 326–334.

Skinner, R. (2015, June). *Critical psychology, indigenous psychology and the "Fitra."* Paper presented at Islamic Psychology and Mental Health: Working Collaboratively, London.

Slife, B. D. (2004). Theoretical challenges to therapy practice and research: The constraint of naturalism. In M. J. Lambert (Ed.), *Bergin and Garfield's handbook of psychotherapy and behavior change* (5th ed., pp. 44–83). New York: Wiley.

Slife, B. D., & Williams, R. N. (1995). *What's behind the research? Discovering hidden assumptions in the behavioral sciences.* Thousand Oaks, CA: Sage. http://dx.doi.org/10.4135/9781483327372

Sperry, L. & Shafranske, E. (2005). *Spiritually Oriented Psychotherapy.* Washington, DC: The American Psychological Association.

Smith, T. B., Bartz, J., & Richards, P. S. (2007). Outcomes of religious and spiritual adaptations to psychotherapy: A meta-analytic review. *Psychotherapy Research*, *17*, 643–655.

Wade, N. G., Worthington, E. L., Jr., & Vogel, D. L. (2007). Effectiveness of religiously tailored interventions in Christian therapy. *Psychotherapy Research*, *17*, 91–105. http://dx.doi.org/10.1080/10503300500497388

Ward, C. (2017). Elucidating the psychospiritual conflict of worldviews and moving towards an indigenous Islamic psychology. In Ahmed, F. J. (Ed.), *Islamic ethics and psychology*. (pp. 49-77). Doha, Qatar: Hamad bin Khalifa University Press.

Worthington, E. L., Jr., Hook, J. N., Davis, D. E., & McDaniel, M. A. (2011). Religion and spirituality. In J. C. Norcross (Ed.), *Relationships that work* (2nd ed., pp. 402–419). New York: New York University Press. http://dx.doi.org/10.1093/acprof:oso/9780199737208.003.0020

Worthington, E. L., Jr., Kurusu, T. A., McCollough, M. E., & Sanders, S. J. (1996). Empirical research on religion and psychotherapeutic processes and outcomes: A 10-year review and research prospectus. *Psychological Bulletin*, *119*, 448–487.

Worthington, E. L., Jr., & Sandage, S. J. (2001). Religion and spirituality. *Psychotherapy: Theory, research, practice, training*, *38*, 473–478. http:// dx.doi.org/10.1037/0033-3204.38.4.473

York, C. (2001). *The effects of ruqya on a non-Muslim: A multiple case study exploration*. Doctoral dissertation, Institute for Transpersonal Psychology, Sofia University, Palo Alto, CA.

York Al-Karam, C. (2015). *Complementary and alternative medicine in psychology: An Islamic therapy for non-Muslims*. In York Al-Karam, C & Haque, A. *Mental health and psychological practice in the United Arab Emirates*. (pp. 169–178). London: Palgrave Macmillan.

York Al-Karam, C. (2017). *Islamic psychology: Defining a discipline*. Background Paper for seminar at the Center for Islamic Legislation and Ethics. https://www.cilecenter.org/en/news/call-papers-islamic-psychology-defining-discipline/

CHAPTER I

An Islamic Theoretical Orientation to Psychotherapy

Abdallah Rothman, LPC

MUCH OF WHAT has been written on and explored with regards to the intersection of Islam and psychology tends to examine the Muslim experience and how psychotherapy can cater to this population. It has been more of a response to the increasing call for multicultural capacity building than it has been an exploration of psychology from the perspective of an Islamic worldview. This focus tends to result in studies of best practice in working with Muslim clients, which can be problematic given that the world's population of Muslims consists of hundreds of different cultures (Kettani, 2010). Yet the desire for the field of psychology to understand how to work with Muslims and the palatable need for mental health services among many populations of Muslim people have given rise to a growing field of Muslim Mental Health. It may be that the most effective way to find common ground among this diverse population is to focus more on the Islamic orientation of these people rather than their relative identity as Muslims. However, there remains a dearth of collective understanding on how an Islamic worldview can be practically and effectively integrated into psychotherapy as well as a lack of understanding of how an Islamic orientation to psychology might also have something to offer to a broader range of people beyond those who identify as Muslim.

I am Muslim and I am a psychotherapist, but I do not consider what I do to be Muslim Mental Health primarily. While many of my clients are Muslim and I work with them on issues of mental health, this label does not accurately describe the focus of my work. My approach to psychology and mental health is based in the Islamic tradition, and Muslims thus tend to identify with it because it is a familiar framework to them. However, when I work with non-Muslim clients I do not change my fundamental orientation, nor do I shift the focus of the actual treatment goals. My goal is to help human beings attune to what works for optimizing their human experience.

I like to make a distinction between Muslim psychology and Islamic psychology. Muslim psychology focuses on how Muslims think and behave. It is primarily a culturally adapted approach to Western therapy that incorporates language, customs, and culturally relevant sentiments into the therapeutic process. This can be useful for many reasons, as it allows for psychotherapy to be more relevant to Muslim populations and to perhaps make such services palatable where they may otherwise be stigmatized as "Western," "secular," "un-Islamic," or simply not culturally relevant. A great number of practitioners are Muslim and have studied psychology and therefore may be equipped to approach their work from within their cultural or religious viewpoint for the benefit of their Muslim clients. Far fewer practitioners have an understanding of how to approach psychotherapy from within an Islamic paradigm of psychology. Thus, this is the distinction between a Muslim psychologist and a Muslim who practices Islamic psychology.

In my understanding, Islamic psychology is an indigenous approach to the study and understanding of human psychology that is informed by the teaching and knowledge from the Quran and the Prophetic tradition (Haque, 1998; Utz, 2011). It is grounded in the ontological paradigm that is elucidated in the Islamic tradition, rather than the secular Western paradigm in which conventional psychology is rooted. Stemming from this, Islamic psychotherapy is an indigenous approach to mental health practice that is derived from Islamic traditions and practices. An Islamic psychology approach to therapy recognizes and engages the soul in the conceptualization of the self and often focuses on the heart rather than the mind as the center of the person. These are just some basic underpinnings that constitute an Islamic theoretical orientation.

As practitioners, when we are trained in theoretical orientations that are based in secular conceptualizations of the human condition that do not necessarily include a recognition of the existence of a higher power, much less any specific understanding of the person in relation to God, we are left to our own devices to incorporate these conceptions into our work with clients. While this may seem straightforward, it can wind up being a patched-together, integrative approach to therapy and not an overt theoretical orientation. What often happens as a result is that clinicians rely on the theoretical orientations in which they have been trained and that operate under a Western secular paradigm as the base of their therapeutic modalities. While many of the techniques, methods, and approaches have merit and offer useful tools for working with clients effectively, the theoretical underpinnings of such orientations are not necessarily aligned with the Islamic paradigm. This can be problematic in working with Muslim clients in that the therapist may be inadvertently guiding them in a direction other than the one defined in the Islamic tradition. What perhaps gets even less attention is the awareness of the possibility that conventional secular conceptualizations of the self may in fact be guiding people in general, not just Muslims, away from the most holistic and optimal way for personal transformation and healing.

Because there is often no clear understanding as to what exactly someone means when they refer to "Islamic psychology," as well as there not being much of a history of the discipline to refer to, I will give a brief account of how my personal journey led me to this approach. I also discuss my experience and how it informs my own interpretation of how to approach an Islamic model of psychotherapy that I have learned from mentors in this emerging field and other teachers grounded in the Islamic tradition. One of the key aspects to my approach to Islamic psychotherapy involves my own deep inner work on myself. I will explain how much of my approach to working with clients stems from and is influenced by my submission to the same journey of self-reflection and self-development on which I am inviting my own clients to embark. I then discuss how this informs my practice, and I provide examples of what methods and techniques I use in my clinical work. I end the chapter with some recommendations for further avenues toward an Islamically integrated approach to psychotherapy.

Development of a Theoretical Orientation

Much of what conventional psychology has become is strictly about studying the brain, behavior, and attributes of the human being that are tangible and measurable—a realm of study that leaves very little room for something like the soul (Reed, 1997). Yet the concept of soul is literally embedded within the original concept of psychology, as the word itself means "study of the psyche." When I first started studying psychology I was not Muslim, but I was fascinated by the idea of the development of the whole self, including the soul. For that reason I was intuitively drawn to humanistic psychology, a subfield that focuses on the whole person and the process of self-actualization, which is the process of working toward realization and maximization of potential (Schneider, Pierson, & Bugental, 2014). My grandfather Leonard Schneider, along with his teacher Abraham Maslow and colleague Fritz Perls, were some of the pioneers of humanistic psychology. In one of the last conversations I had with my grandfather before he died, he told me that he wished he would have paid more attention to religion and spiritual traditions and how they can be of great use within the therapeutic encounter for providing structure to people's understanding of themselves and their own personal growth. I was intrigued by this notion and made it the focus of my investigation in my own study of psychology. I saw myself as continuing my grandfather's work where he had left off.

In addition to my study of psychology, I was actively involved in the study of various religious traditions. I was as eclectic in my theoretical approach to psychology as I was in my theological approach to spirituality: I couldn't bring myself to commit to just one path. In my early career, I often claimed to have an "eclectic" orientation, which in the field of psychotherapy is often seen as a cop-out. Similarly, with regard to spirituality and religion, I claimed to be spiritual but not religious. I studied and admired all religions and incorporated aspects of them into my own personal path but did not subscribe to a religion, or even perhaps the idea of religion. Like some who are turned off by or skeptical of conventional notions of God but consider themselves spiritual, my sense was that there was a universal power that connects all living things.

Whereas some people tend to reject the idea of God in opposition to how God is portrayed, I was comfortable with the idea that there are many different ways to understand and relate to the spiritual, Divine Reality. My own feeling is that what I call God is in essence the same thing as what another may describe in other terms. Therefore, belief in God was never a question for me. I liked to quote Carl Jung (1977) in my answer to whether I believed in God by saying, "I do not believe, I know" (p. 429) To me, the existence of God was a given, and I believed that our task in this life is to become closer to God, which I interpreted as what self-actualization really was: God-consciousness. Essentially, my relationship to psychology was infused with my spiritual journey.

With the last words of my grandfather in my mind, coupled with my own experiences with religious spiritual devotion, I came to the acute realization that without a dedicated path I was hitting a glass ceiling in my own growth. I came to see that I could not advance further on my path of personal growth unless I committed to a path that disciplined me to allow for deeper transformation and expansion of consciousness by working through my psychological imbalances in a systematic and successive way. The eclectic approach to both a theoretical orientation to psychology as well as to a theological orientation to spirituality suffers from lack of structure and theoretical grounding that is situated within one paradigm. This can result in elusive, unclear stances that, in the realm of the unseen—the soul or psyche—can become limiting at best, if not dangerous. I eventually determined that in order to continue on my inner quest I needed to commit to a path. This was simultaneously true of my approach to psychotherapy and my personal spiritual discipline. Thus, my ultimate landing on a theoretical orientation to psychology is inextricably linked to my eventual embracing of a religious path. In fact, the two were one and the same.

Approaching Islam as Psychology, Psychology as Islam

In my search for a path that would primarily orient me toward spiritual self-development, I discovered a deeply intricate science to the conceptualization of the soul, and it was grounded in Islam. Given the way in which I came to embrace it, there is very little separation for me between Islam as a religion and psychology/psychotherapy as different disciplines that I am adapting or integrating with Islam. For me, the spiritual work and the psychological work are inextricably interconnected. I see Islam as a psychology and believe that psychology (the study of the psyche) can be realized fully through the Islamic tradition. I do not consider what I do as an integration of Islam into psychotherapy as much as I consider my practice of psychotherapy as a translation of concepts relating to the soul and to healing from the Islamic tradition into the language of psychology within a therapeutic process.

My training in Western psychotherapy gave me access to a wonderful tool kit of approaches to counseling clients—for example, techniques of engaging clients in self-reflection, skills of active listening, and therapeutic techniques that elicit clients to open up in order to gain access to their inner process and thus be better positioned to help guide them toward treatment goals. The treatment goals, however, in my approach to psychotherapy from an Islamic paradigm are different from the Western conceptualization of therapy and therefore need to be reoriented in order to use those techniques and skills in Islamic psychotherapy.

Unlike some Western approaches to therapy, my goal is not necessarily to get the client to where they want to be, as that is not as important as them wanting what is best for them. It says in the Quran, "You may hate a thing and it is good for you; and you may love a thing and it is bad for you. And Allah Knows, while you know not" (2:216). From an Islamic perspective, "Allah is the best of Planners" (8:30), and He is the One who knows what is best for us. So from this approach it is fundamentally a very different paradigm that determines what the goal of therapy is. To be clear, physical symptoms and severe mental illness often should be treated with medicine under supervision of an appropriate medical psychiatric practitioner. However, from an Islamic paradigm of psychology, most sicknesses of the heart and soul are seen as a result of the person being disconnected from God (Ghazali, 1986), while others are seen as challenges or tests that people need to go through in order to purify their soul, and may not in fact actually be curable or need to be fully eradicated Thus, an Islamic approach to psychotherapy can often help reframe clients' struggles in light of spiritual growth, regardless of a client's particular beliefs, and can often work well in tandem with medical interventions.

The Islamic tradition is a rich source within which healing and therapeutic techniques and interventions can be found. It is an exhaustive medicine cabinet of remedies for every ailment of the soul. My job as therapist is to be a creative pharmacist, choosing different combinations of Islamic soul medicine to fit the client's current situation and need in a way that makes sense to his or her mind and heart. It is a process of translating wisdom from the Islamic tradition into practical deliverable action items that speak to the person where they are and for what they are currently struggling with. It is similar to what an Imam or a *shaykh* (spiritual guide) might do, but my emphasis is more on making it relevant to clients' personal and emotional struggles and studying and understanding who they are and what will make sense to them rather than focusing primarily on the solution itself as an overarching truth. For this reason, it is important that the therapist have knowledge of relevant Islamic teachings in order to inform the treatment. They must know what Islam says about principles of the self and, for working with Muslim clients, have some basic knowledge of *fard al ayn* (individual religious obligations) as those are related to the remedies of the soul.

My Islamic theoretical orientation aims to understand a client's situation from the viewpoint of the *fitrah* (natural disposition) of the human soul. Without projecting my religious beliefs onto them, which would be both unethical and un-Islamic, I can help clients reflect on what course of action is more congruent with their own internal moral compass, their own *fitrah*. When the solution to the problem really relies on a specific determination of what Islamic law says about it—for instance, in cases of marriage and divorce—this is where it is essential to have partnerships with Imams in the local community, as I do in my own practice, to consult on cases that require an Islamic *fiqh* perspective as appropriate according to the orientation of the client. I have also done the same in working with clients of different faiths by referring them to their own religious leaders. This gives an opportunity for therapists to educate Imams or other faith leaders on ideas of mental health and best counseling practice, which allows for an alliance that is an ideal model that I feel should be the exemplary goal for the developing field of Islamic psychology.

My Practice

My spiritual practice is central to my practice of psychotherapy. My own self-development work in my own life informs and is the primary mechanism I use in working with clients. I operate under the notion that God is the true healer and it is really only He that can guide a person and change their heart, a sentiment shared by many traditional healing philosophies (Kiev, 1964; Moodley & West, 2005). Since my job is to be a conduit for that connection to God, the best thing I can do to be an effective practitioner is to "get out of the way" (Duffy & Veltri, 1998). The more I can clean my own heart, the more God can give to the client what they need. I do this by constantly keeping up with my own *jihad an nafs* (struggle against the lower self) and thus modeling this for the client.

People tend to take guidance easiest from those who are living examples, as it is more relatable. The power in this is similar to the idea of transference in that people have a natural inclination or need to identify with another person and see him- or herself in that person as a reflection (Jung, 2013). I use my humanness as a tool for connecting with the client and being a reflection of their humanness. I make an effort to recognize that I too am growing as a result of the therapeutic relationship. I often find that my clients mirror my own personal struggles with the issues they present in session. In relationship, we come face-to-face with ourselves, and in these human struggles we have access to come closer to God, not just through spiritual transcendence.

This was the blessing of the Prophet Mohammed (peace and blessing upon him [pbuh]) in that he was sent as a living human example of how to be in this world in the best of ways. He embodied the qualities of a psychologically balanced person who lived in accordance with *fitrah*. Therefore, we have in his example both a model for the therapist and the client. Whereas the Prophet (pbuh) was believed to have a perfected character, we all are imperfect and it is known and expected that we make mistakes. I make it clear to my clients that the goal is only that we aim toward this ideal in order to work on healing ourselves, not that we hold ourselves up to such unattainably high standards. Looking to the Prophetic example acts as a guiding light that shows us the extent of our potential for growth, so that we have hope and aspiration to improve, not to attain perfection, but simply to continue striving toward it.

The character of the Prophet Mohammed (pbuh) is reported to have been a perfect example of unbounded love and positive regard toward others. As he said, "None of you are true believers until you love for your fellow human beings what you love for yourself" (*Sahih al-Bukhari* 13.6). One of the most well-known concepts to come out of the humanistic psychology movement is the Rogerian concept of the therapist having "unconditional positive regard" for the client because it creates the container necessary for the client to begin to open up to the difficult process of therapy (Rogers, 1966). Just as you cannot truly be a believer without this condition of love, similarly you cannot truly operate from within an Islamic paradigm without reflecting love for your client. The distinction between the love of God (*Al Wadud*) that the Prophet was reflecting and that of the Rogerian concept of "unconditional" love or positive regard is that while this deep love is given to all generously, it may not be accurate to say that it is "unconditional." The Prophet balanced his unbounded love with firm resolve in standing in the truth, and he lovingly guided people toward what is better for them (Lings, 1995). Thus, an Islamic paradigm approach requires a compassionate, merciful stance that simultaneously stands firm in the notion that it is not potentially in the client's best interest to do something that is harmful for his or her soul.

The eleventh-century Islamic scholar Abu Hamid Al Ghazali was a key figure in helping elucidate how to conceptualize the self or soul in an Islamic paradigm, and he provided the foundations for an Islamic model of the self/soul as outlined in the Quran. Ghazali described four key aspects of the soul of the human being; the *nafs* (lower self), the *qalb* (heart), the *aql* (cognition), and the *ruh* (spirit). All of these aspects have unique attributes and mechanisms that make up the inner working of the human soul. However, the distinctions are mostly for our benefit in understanding the structure and function of the human condition; in reality they are all one integrated whole, and therefore these words are often used interchangeably in reference to the aspects of the person. The primary utility in understanding these distinct functions of the self is in the work of *tazkiyat an nafs* (purification of the self) and in turn Islamic psychotherapy, in that they provide a useful guide to assessment and treatment. Consequently, many practitioners of Islamic psychology in the developing of the field and indigenous therapeutic approaches have used this model in conceptualizations of therapeutic interventions (for example, Skinner, 2010; Keshavarzi & Haque, 2013).

I use these four aspects to organize some examples of how I work with clients at different levels, or entry points, in the process of therapy. I should mention that this organization is somewhat arbitrary and designed for the purpose of explaining it more clearly in a relatively linear fashion, which lends itself better to the written word. In reality, the process is much more fluid and interconnected, as is the nature of the human being and the art of therapy. In addition, the process of self-growth is neither linear nor sequential. There are stages of the *nafs*'s development as it goes through the process of reformation—namely, *nafs-al-ammarah* (commanding self; 12:53), *nafs-al-awwamah* (reproaching self; 75:2), and *nafs-al-mutmainnah* (contented self; 89:27), which are successive in the transcendence from the lower self (*nafs*) to the higher self (*ruh*) that is more in line with *fitrah*. A person is subject to cycle in and out of these stages as he or she engages in the struggle with his or her *nafs*. Although one may achieve growth, remaining at that stage is not guaranteed nor static, as the *nafs* is in a constant state of flux, thus requiring constant diligence on the part of the person who is engaged in this developmental process.

This is where my work with clients is, in keeping them engaged in the process, attuned to their self and equipped with the tools necessary to make advancements on the path. Within this process there are several tools at my disposal, most of which are directly from the source of the Islamic tradition and the practice of *tazkiyat an nafs*, with some knowledge and techniques from Western psychotherapy and other disciplines that I incorporate in the process of integrating knowledge to increase the effectiveness of the approach and make sure it lands with each client.

I now explain some of the techniques and interventions that I use in my process within the therapeutic encounter. This is not an exhaustive list, as a great many tools are at our disposal within the Islamic tradition, but these are ones that I use quite often in my own psycho-spiritual practice and are central to my practice of Islamic psychotherapy. For the sake of clarity and organization, the following interventions are categorized relative to the four levels of the self (*qalb, aql, nafs, ruh*).

Interventions

Qalb

Centering in the Heart. One of the primary techniques I use with all my clients is first and foremost to orient them to the *qalb* (heart) as the center of the self. Most of us are more oriented to our minds as we identify with our thoughts, beliefs, and cognitive constructs. While the mind is necessary and useful in the process of therapy, it is not my main focus. I can spend a great deal of time helping someone to clear their thoughts and/or change their way of thinking, but if we don't address the place in the person's heart that is the emotional source of those thoughts, there won't be real transformation and it often will not last. According to the Islamic model of the self, the *qalb* is the center of the human being and thus is where much of the focus of Islamic psychology centers (Inayat, 2005; Skinner, 2010, 2018; Keshavarzi & Haque, 2013).

A famous *hadith qudsi* (words of Allah expressed in the Prophet's words) says, "Neither My earth nor My heavens can contain Me, but the heart of a believing servant contains Me." This does not mean that God is manifested in His creation, as that would be counter to the central Islamic concept of *tawhid* (oneness of God). It simply means that the *qalb* is the access point in which we are able to connect directly with the Divine. It is the same place where people often attribute intuition or a sense of knowing what is right; as the common expressions, say, "I know it in my heart," or "Follow your heart." The *qalb* is the center of the self and is where we are able to connect to our *fitrah*, our true, pure self that came from God and will ultimately return to God. If we attune to this heart center constantly, we can align with our *fitrah* more consistently and raise our level of *taqwa* (God-consciousness).

A popular hadith (authenticated saying of the Prophet) says, "Surely, in the body there is a small piece of flesh; if it is sound, the whole body is sound, and if it is corrupted, the whole body is corrupted, and that is surely the heart" (Bukhari). The *qalb* is sound when it is living in accordance with its *fitrah*, in awareness of and alignment with God, which then affects the state of the whole person. The *qalb* is corrupted when it gets filled with things other than God and forgets and becomes out of accord with its *fitrah*. Living in the *dunya* (temporal world), our experience is that of individual self-identification and separation from other life and God, rather than an awareness of *tawhid* (unity). This experience of the temporal world can veil our true self and distract us from a *fitrah* way of being and leads us to become preoccupied with our outward persona's and the identity of the self that we project to others in our worldly lives. Especially in societies dominated by the Western paradigm, which is influenced by the Cartesian assertion "*Cogito ergo sum*" (I think therefore I am), our tendency is to connect our identity with our thoughts. This is reflected in the significant cognitive emphases within theories of identity in Western social psychology, such as social identity theory / self-categorization theory (Tajfel & Turner, 1979, 1985; Turner et al., 1987) and identity process theory (Breakwell, 1986; Jaspal & Breakwell, 2014). Thus, one of my first tasks in orienting my clients toward an Islamic understanding of the self is to teach them how to center their awareness in their *qalb*, in their heart, and move away from the tendency to overidentify with the mind.

One of the ways I do this is by introducing visualization and breathing practices as part of the therapeutic treatment. In session I use visualization to help clients bring their conscious awareness to the physical place in their body where their heart center is—in the chest. I usually ask them to bow their head to their chest and to imagine that they are relinquishing their overidentification with the mind's chatter and allowing for the heart to take more of a center stage during this process. I also frequently use metaphors to embody this shift in awareness. Using diaphragm breathing techniques that I teach them in session, which are similar to that of Buddhist meditation (Hanh, 2016) and Hindu *pranayama* (Saraswati, & Hiti 1996) and have been shown to have significant health benefits (Jerath, Edry, Barnes, & Jerath, 2006) but that are derived from within Islamic spiritual traditions, I ask them to pay close attention to the process of breathing. I guide them to bring their awareness to the process of filling their lungs with air and exhaling, and the awareness of the fact that where this is happening, in the lungs, is the same place as the heart center. I ask the client to envision the incoming air as light and explain the concept of *bast* (expansion) as it relates to the hadith of the Prophet (pbuh) in reference to the *ayah* in the Quran that states, "one whose breast God has expanded to (accept) Islam, he is upon a light from his Lord" (39:22). When asked by one of the companions what is the meaning of expanding in the context of this *ayah*, the Prophet (pbuh) said, "It is enlarging, for, when the light is cast into the heart, the chest is enlarged and expanded for it" (Ibn Mas'ud). The technique is usually introduced after the first few sessions and is revisited throughout the course of therapy. This process helps slow a person down and connect with the true center of one's self. It is also a tool to counteract anxiety, opening a door of access to the place in the person where emotional material is stored. While I will only do this type of connecting to the heart in session after building trust and safety with clients, I do give them more simple centering and breathing exercises to do on their own outside of session as a self-regulating practice.

When a person feels any type of emotion, whether love, fear, or anxiety, there is usually a corresponding visceral response in the heart. Most people are familiar with the sensation of getting "butterflies" when they are nervous or a sense of *qabd* (contraction), or constricting in the chest, when experiencing anxiety. These are signs of the emotional material that is located in the *qalb* and that correspond to feelings. Whenever we have an experience that serves to disconnect us from the love and contentment that comes from an acute awareness of God's reality, whether in the form of an animalistic impulse from our lower urges or simply entering a state of *ghafla* (forgetting God) induced by internal or external factors, such as trauma, our hearts harden little by little. In a *sahih hadith* (authentic saying of the Prophet), the Prophet (pbuh) explains, in reference to the *ayah* (verse) in the Quran that describes the rust, stain, or covering on the heart (83:14), that we acquire "black spots" on our hearts from transgressions that in turn need to be cleaned or removed by making *tawbah* (turning back to God); (Tirmidhī 3334). These black spots that accumulate on the heart over time are an inevitable part of living in the duality and separation from God that is characteristic of life in the *dunya*, and not necessarily a result of our own faults. If we do not tend to them and clear them, our whole heart can become encrusted or covered over to the point that we are completely veiled from God and live in a constant state of separation, where we only identify with our externally projected self and the temporal world and essentially become hardhearted. From the perspective of someone who does not believe in God, this can be experienced as being disconnected from a sense of purity and purpose. Some relative version of this phenomenon is generally what is at the root of many ills of the soul or mental health issues, and, as prescribed by the Prophet in the hadith referenced above, one of the best remedies for this is the act of *tawbah*.

Tawbah. *Tawbah* is sometimes defined as "forgiveness." However, it is a concept that is more integrally related to the heart than what is often understood in the concept of forgiveness. This is exemplified in the fact that the root of the word *qalb* means to turn, so the heart turns this way or that, and *tawbah* means "to turn toward God." So *tawbah* is the process of turning our hearts toward the Divine presence, bringing our inner self into witnessing and accessing that primordial source. *Tawbah* is an integral part of the practice within the Islamic paradigm and it is mentioned thirty-five times in the Quran. Throughout the Quran, it is explained that God is oft forgiving and that we should continually come to Him asking for forgiveness, no matter how great or how plentiful are our sins, even if they amount to all of the bubbles in the sea foam of all the oceans of the earth (Bukhari 1410). In the Islamic paradigm, this concept of forgiveness is similar to the Western psychological concept that releasing oneself from holding on to feelings of guilt can lift a burden from the psyche of the individual and positively affect mental health (McCullough & Witvliet, 2002). However, *tawbah* is not exclusively about guilt as a result of transgression. The Prophet is said to have made *tawbah* one hundred times a day (Muslim 42), and he was believed to be free from sin. Thus, this aspect of turning toward Allah is the central mechanism that enables one to find a similar release experienced in forgiveness. Yet it is more of a release from the disharmony that is caused from existing in a state of individuation, separate from, or rather unconscious of, one's connectedness to God. *Tawbah* is so central to the Islamic paradigm that out of the ninety-nine names of Allah, four are related to forgiveness. One of those names, or attributes, is *Al Afuw* (the eliminator of sins), which indicates that in God's supreme mercy we have the opportunity to be completely free of all remnants of our sins, transgressions, and slip-ups. Thus we truly have the potential to be free from these black spots on our hearts and achieve a clean *qalb* and a pure state, not just the potential to be better or happier than before but to potentially transcend and elevate our inner state of being as a result of witnessing God's *tawhid*.

Tawbah is not about beating ourselves up over our mistakes, nor is it about dwelling in feelings of guilt. I often need to spend time reframing and restructuring for my Muslim clients to correct their relationship to this Islamic principle, especially for those clients who carry burdens of guilt. *Istighfar* (asking for forgiveness) is not about dwelling on the wrong that was committed, as the conception of "sin" or "transgression" is not always about a wrong act. Between the two *khutbahs* (sermons) in *salat al jummah* (Muslim Friday prayer), the reason that the Imam sits down for such a short time in *istighfar* is that we are not supposed to dwell on our sins, as God knows what we have done, as do we, and the idea is not to bring greater attention to the act but to bring attention to the remembrance of God. Thus, *tawbah* should be invoked not only for major transgressions but even for more subtle things, such as simply forgetting God. *Tawbah* really is about returning to our true self, as the root of the Arabic word *tawab* means "to return." It's about recognizing our reliance on God and recentering our focus on the greater reality of our existence over the distractions within our *nafs* (self) and the *dunya*.

The way I use *tawbah* in therapy mostly takes the form of this latter aspect of returning to God, rather than asking for forgiveness from major transgressions. For example, a client comes in with the presenting problem of loss of appetite and sleep deprivation due to increased anxiety, and in unpacking the underlying issue, we discover that he is preoccupied with the worry that he will lose his job. In processing his feelings and thoughts about the situation, he continues to focus on his boss and the potential that she has to fire him, which in turn increases his sense of powerlessness as he feels anxious about his boss potentially making a decision that will greatly impact his life and means of sustenance. He feels out of control. His visceral feeling of anxiety is centered in his chest, in the heart center, which has created a sense of *qabd* (constriction). After teaching him to center in the heart, I would guide him to make *tawbah* into the same place in his heart, the specific location in his chest, where he feels the constriction. The objective is twofold: to reconnect his heart to the remembrance of God and return (*tawab*) to Him and to restructure the way he thinks about the situation by correcting the cognition that attributes his destiny to the decision of his boss and replacing it with the cognition that is in line with the Islamic paradigm that acknowledges that Allah is *Ar Razaq* (the provider). The client is guided to make *tawbah* because he has forgotten that Allah is the one who controls his provision, not his boss. In addition to reciting the words *astaghfirallah* in the heart, we may even repeat the name *Ar Razaq* to bring the awareness of that quality of God into his heart. This is the practice of *dhikr* (remembrance); as the Quran says, "Surely in the remembrance of Allah do hearts find rest" (13:28), and is something I use at all levels of the self. The cognitive restructuring part, however, is the domain of the *aql*.

Aql

Cognitive Restructuring (Islamic cognitive behavioral therapy). Cognitive behavioral therapy (CBT) is one of the most popular methods in modern therapy. This is due to the ease with which it can be standardized and measured, its solution-focused treatment, and its concentration on the thoughts of the mind as the main strategy for meeting therapeutic treatment goals (Cuijpers et al., 2014; Hans & Hiller, 2013; Stewart & Chambless, 2009). While the Islamic model is more concerned with the heart than the mind as the central focus of intervention, cognitive restructuring certainly has its place within the Islamic paradigm. Over one thousand years before the advent of CBT, the ninth-century Muslim scholar Abu Zayd al-Balkhi wrote a treatise (Badri, 2013; Awaad & Ali, 2015, 2016) that specifically details the same phenomena and processes that are now lauded over by the Western domain of psychology as CBT. Along with his work on identifying many of the diagnoses of psychopathology used today, al-Balkhi recognized the importance of restructuring cognitions to align with values and bringing the mind into the process of healing the soul and integrating worship of God.

The process of CBT involves the restructuring of maladaptive thoughts and replacing them with cognitions that are more constructive toward the treatment goal of the patient (Beck, 1976; Dobson, 2009; Ellis, 1962). The constructive cognitions can be catered to the belief system of the patient to work toward the achievement of congruence with his or her individual self-concept. Thus, one aspect of an Islamic CBT approach is that it can play an important role in finding power and motivation toward clients' goals by putting things into the context of their belief system. This technique can also be helpful in working with Muslim clients whose presenting problem or underlying issue may be rooted in a misunderstanding of a religious belief and can thus be corrected through appropriate education to change the problematic belief or cognition.

Carrying on from the example above, the next step after orienting the client's *qalb* toward reliance on God would be to correct the belief that the client's boss has the power to change his destiny and keep him from earning money. The orientation within the Islamic paradigm is that God is the only one with the power to give or take away a person's job, God is the One who provides *rizq* (sustenance)—including but not limited to money—and God is the best of Planners whose wisdom and mercy is in everything that He ordains. Thus, the goal is to restructure the client's cognitive construct to include these notions, trust that God has a plan that is better than the client's, and that the objective is to submit to that divine plan. Or in the case that the person does not have an overt orientation to the idea of the will of God in this way, we would focus on the notion that our personal agency only goes as far as the things within our control and that by recognizing and accepting that many things are out of our control, we can reduce unwanted anxiety. I would only do this, however, after listening compassionately and validating the client's feelings. Eventually I would bring the client's awareness to the way he or she is perceiving the situation and help hold that up against his or her own personal values in relation to this principle. This process does not work effectively in isolation. Rather, I use this strategy in conjunction with others mentioned here, and this is a constant process of reorienting thoughts, something that I teach the client to do habitually. Another cognitive strategy that can help reinforce the changing of thought patterns is the use of *dhikr* (remembrance).

Dhikr. The practice of *dhikr*, or remembrance, in essence, is an act of reorienting one's awareness toward a deeper truth than the temporal reality we are generally focused on in our daily lives. As mentioned, I use *dhikr* at every level of the self, as it is a central tool in orienting the client back to one's *fitrah* and reconnecting with the primordial source. Whereas using *dhikr* at the level of the *qalb* is to open the person's heart to receive God's mercy and bring the remembrance into a deeper internal unconscious place inside the self where the pain of disconnection has left black spots, the use of *dhikr* at the level of the *aql* is to reorient a client's conscious thoughts toward remembrance of God. This practice is similar to the use of mantras in the Hindu and Buddhist traditions, in that the person repeats a phrase over and over again that can become somewhat meditative (Ashley-Farrand, 2008). Whereas I sometimes use *dhikr* in this way—perhaps out loud in session with clients to calm them if they are having an anxiety attack, for example—the way I use it more often at the level of the *aql* is as assigned homework outside of a session.

Based on the particular cognition that may be resulting in problematic feelings or behaviors, I help the client devise an appropriate phrase of *dhikr* either from those prescribed by the Prophet Mohammed (pbuh), or something else that is relative to the context. This is to counteract the incessant negative thoughts that often become habitual responses to experiences based on cognitive constructs. The mind has a natural tendency to perseverate on things that can often wind up being negative thoughts, as positive ones tend to require more conscious effort (Seligman, 2004). Therefore, an individual must be diligent about consciously inserting positive statements in the mind to counteract the negative. The popular positive psychology movement (Seligman, 2004; Lopez, Pedrotti, & Snyder, 2014) recognizes this, as did al-Balkhi when he recommended that one should keep positive thoughts on hand to use when needed, just as one might keep medicines in a medicine cabinet (Haque, 2004; Badri, 2013).

To give an example, a client is struggling with feelings of inadequacy. Through exploring what triggers these feelings, we uncover a consistent tendency for her to compare herself to other women in social situations. This mental comparison takes on the form of a narrative that she is not as good as these other woman and that she doesn't deserve to be happy—that she is unlovable. As part of my treatment with her, in addition to processing the historic events in her life that formulated these cognitions, and uncovering the places in her *qalb* where the unconscious material is stored, I would develop a strategy with her to deconstruct the thought pattern that holds these cognitions in place. Recognizing the fact that the mind needs to dwell on thoughts or phrases, I would give her new statements or phrases to replace the maladaptive ones. Within the Islamic tradition, several phrases can be implemented in this way. The ninety-nine names of Allah that each focus on a specific attribute can target a certain need. Additionally, I may recommend *astaghfirallah* (forgive me God), *salawat* (praises) on the Prophet, *Allahu Akbar* (God is the greatest), *subhanallah* (glory to God), or even simply just repeating the word "Allah," which I recommend to Muslim clients often as a place to start as it can be the most familiar and directly effective. For non-Muslims, I often recommend repeating the word "love" as a way of reminding them of the universal energy of love that is available to all and to orient them toward generating this concept within him- or herself. In this case, I would instruct the client to use some of the techniques that we have worked on in session to bring awareness to herself and awareness to her thoughts and to notice when these maladaptive negative thoughts arise (Beck, 1976; Dobson, 2009; Ellis, 1962). At those moments, she should practice making a habit of simply saying, for instance, the word "Allah" silently in her mind on top of, after, or instead of the thoughts we are trying to counteract. She can integrate this with some of the breathing practices as well as the awareness of the heart center, to bring her awareness back to Allah's love and acceptance of her. As with all of the interventions I use, they interconnect with other methods and other levels of the self. In this case particularly, in conjunction with the implementation of *dhikr*, I would work with the client at the *nafs* level to become aware of herself and her tendencies, preferences, and urges.

Nafs

Muhasabah. Muhasabah is the practice of taking account of the self, an inventory of the *nafs*. While it involves bringing awareness to the whole integrated self (*qalb, aql, nafs, ruh*), often the focus is on the specific aspect of the lower self as this is the aspect that most needs to be worked on and reformed. The term *nafs* is often used to represent the part of the person that most closely resembles the ego in Western psychology. One of the main differences between the concept of the ego and that of the *nafs* is that in the Islamic paradigm the *nafs* is not considered to be bad in and of itself and can be trained to serve the whole. The *nafs* is influenced by the *hawa* (desire), which is a function of the lower self and its drives and urges that lead us toward indulgence in self-satisfaction. These inclinations are natural, but if allowed to run wild they will lead us toward an existence that is mired in the external world and separate from a life of *taqwa* (God-consciousness). But if we put them in check by striving to control our lower urges, then we can rise above the powerful hold they can have on us and thus master our *nafs* to serve our higher self or soul.

In explaining this dynamic and our part in it when working with my clients, I like to put a spin on the ancient Greek Delphic maxim, *Gnothi seauton* (Know thyself), and say that we must "no thyself." What I mean is that in order to truly know oneself in the Islamic concept of *fitrah* is to say "no" to ourselves, to limit our desires and rein in our thoughts, feelings, and behaviors. Within the Islamic tradition, this process is known as *tahdhīb al-akhlāq* (refinement of character) and involves the process of disciplining the lower tendencies of the *nafs* and bringing our thoughts, intentions, and actions in alignment with the Prophetic example, as the Prophet is believed to have been sent to "perfect good character," as the *sahih hadith* reports (Bukhari). The practice of *muhasabah* is a useful tool in this process of the perfection of character that I often use with my clients to bring awareness to their thoughts, intentions, and behavior. However, it is important to first establish the notion of self-love as a foundation upon which this practice can be implemented so as to keep it oriented toward constructive growth rather than destructive self-criticism. The perfection of character is not simply an indulgence for those who are not struggling with more severe presenting problems. Strong reactions to situations, that can be a result of triggering past trauma, often show up as maladaptive responses in the form of "negative" character traits, such as anger for example. That anger may very well be justified and have its place to a degree, but when it is not put into balance it can become destructive and impede a client's ability to heal from the trauma. Thus, bringing awareness to one's reactions provides necessary information for where to focus the process of achieving *i'tidaal* (equilibrium), or coming into balance.

While keeping a journal of self-reflection to help clients bring awareness to their thoughts and behaviors can be very useful for this process, I find that most clients do not follow through with this practice consistently. I therefore am more interested in introducing it as a habit that they can form in their daily life, which they do in the back of their mind, and can integrate into their day-to-day activities. By taking account of our own thoughts and reactions, we can shift the focus from examining other people's behavior in relationships, and projecting irritation on to them, and instead choose to examine our own behavior. In identifying the flaws in others we usually are projecting our own dissatisfaction with ourselves or incongruence with our *fitrah*. This dynamic is what is often at the heart of difficulties within intimate relationships (Berne, 2010) and why in the Islamic tradition marriage is considered to be a significant avenue for working on the self (Maqsood, 1995). Through *muhasabah* we can become more self-aware and cognizant of where we may be out of balance and how our character may be out of line with our own values and those set by the Prophetic example. Once we have this information, we are in a position to make changes. The Quran says, "Allah will not change the condition of a people until they change what is in themselves" (13:11). God can change our state if we turn to Him, but we first must make an effort toward change in ourselves by enacting our will. While this starts with *muhasabah* and the inner *jihad an nafs* in the battle to correct our internal activity of the self, there is also an external aspect that is equally important in order to solidify these changes and manifest them in action. This is where the refinement of character extends beyond modeling just our character on the qualities of the Prophet, but modeling our behavior and habits as well.

Physical *Sunnah*. Once one has an understanding of one's weaknesses and tendencies, it is necessary to follow up that awareness with action. If it stays in the theoretical phase of knowledge without action, it does little good. As they say, "Knowing is half the battle." The other half is actually fighting the battle against the self with discipline; this is the *jihad an nafs*. While *jihad an nafs* is both an internal and an external struggle against our lower self, we often do not connect the two and naively think that, by just being aware of ourselves and knowing our imbalances and tendencies, we can avoid unwanted patterns and thus potential harm. As human beings, it is an absolute imperative to involve our physical being in the process of self-mastery. The outer rules of engagement that are set forth in the Islamic tradition can be seen as a map for navigating the pitfalls and distractions of life in the *dunya*. Physical discipline is key to bringing the body in alignment with the rest of the self to strengthen and empower our capabilities of personal development and psychological growth (Penedo & Dahn, 2005). Within the Islamic tradition, particularly the *sunnah* (ways of being) of the Prophet Mohammed (pbuh) we have a whole artillery of tools at our disposal for warding off temptation and distraction by which the *nafs* is so easily swayed.

In my own practice as well as my practice of therapy with my clients, I invoke specific *sunnat* of the Prophet as daily discipline habits that I believe are essential for establishing constancy and increasing internal balance. These behavioral commitments actualize our *niyyah* (intention) and *aml* (action) and help maintain a connection to the rope of Allah amid the ever-changing state of our *nafs* and the constant ups and downs of life. I myself have a strict routine of physical practices that I do habitually over and above my five daily *fard* (obligatory) prayers. These include fasting two days a week, waking up in the middle of the night for *tahajud* (night prayer), eating halal (permissible) *wa taib* (healthy), daily *nawafl* (optional) prayers, reciting Quran, doing *dhikr*, and exercising. All of these things were the practices of the Prophet (pbuh), which he did specifically to set an example for how human beings can live in the *dunya* in accordance with our *fitrah* for a more successful life. This significant level of commitment is clearly not for everyone. Self-discipline is not an easy thing to maintain. However, given my work as a therapist, I find that it is the only way that I can maintain a clear and clean heart to allow for God to be the true guide, and it also provides the strength, stability, and stamina necessary to work in a deep and meaningful way with clients in navigating the darker parts of themselves. In this profession, it is perhaps more important for the clinicians to make every effort to practice what they preach as maintaining self-awareness becomes an ethical responsibility.

While I do not hold the same expectations of clients as I do of therapists regarding the level and amount of self-discipline practices, I strongly encourage my clients to adopt some of these practices to the level that they can realistically commit to and maintain. While from an Islamic perspective the specific *sunnah* of the Prophet are believed by Muslims to have *baraka* (blessing) in them because they were beloved by the beloved of Allah, there is a lot of room for Muslims and non-Muslims alike to adopt practices that deliver similar results. For instance, there are specific *sunnah* sports that were recommended by the Prophet, namely swimming, wrestling, horseback riding, and archery. Each of these has a certain inherent wisdom and balancing effect for the person who practices them. But in addition, a general benefit results from any physical exercise as it can have profound balancing effects on the whole person (Salmon, 2001). Clients can thus choose activities that fit their own personal *fitrah* or that are more easily accessible to them in order to make it practical and to have longevity. I work with my clients, sometimes in partnership with their doctors or fitness instructors, to construct a bespoke routine toward which they can work.

In addition to these regular habitual practices, I also recommend physical *sunnah* acts as interventions or remedies for specific singular situations to counteract specific destructive character traits with which a person is struggling. Through hadith we learn that the Prophet gave certain behavioral remedies. For example, he said when a person becomes angry, if he is standing he should sit, and if still angry then lie down, and that making *wudu* (ablution) can cool the anger. Also he recommended physical exercise and fasting as a remedy for diminishing sexual passion for unmarried men. While these concepts and behaviors can potentially resonate with believing Muslims, when presented simply as effective prescriptions purely for their practical benefit, I have found them to be just as useful and powerful in treating non-Muslims who do not have the context of reverence for the Prophet or a connection to the Islamic tradition. A great many behavioral remedies within the Islamic tradition provide solutions to many common mental health concerns. Whether treating acute presenting problems or establishing healthy patterns that bring the body and mind into alignment, these tools are foundational in the process of opening the channels to healing by aligning with *fitrah* and thus working toward becoming better versions of ourselves.

Ruh

Muraqaba/Tafakkur. People's relationship to religion can often take on more of a transactional approach than a transformational one. This is a result of being cut off from the *ruh* (spirit), the aspect of the human soul that has direct access to the divine source. While the acquisition of knowledge through studying is one way of learning the deeper meaning in the prescriptions of the *deen* and is greatly encouraged throughout the Quran and hadith, as with other religious scripture, there is also another kind of knowledge that comes directly from God. In the Islamic tradition, this is known as *ma'rifa* (gnosis) and is a key part of psychological well-being because it is the active ingredient in the process of receiving God's *shifaa* (healing) of the soul. While I can help navigate the path for a person to develop the practices and attributes that will bring things into balance by knowing oneself and aligning with one's *fitrah*, only God can truly transform a person's heart. Thus, the work of the *jihad an nafs* (struggle of the self) and of *tazkiyat an nafs* (purification of the self) is all a process of uncovering the crust over our *nafs* to open the channels to connect with and open up to God. This is a unique feature of an Islamic paradigm of human psychology in that it includes an actual mechanism within the self to receive directly from the primordial source.

Muraqaba is sometimes translated as "meditation." However, it is not secluded to the type of mindfulness that often people attribute to that term. As discussed above with the interventions related to the level of *aql*, cognitive awareness certainly has its place in the Islamic paradigm of psychology. *Muraqaba*, however, is more about tuning into our inner self holistically—*qalb*, *aql*, *nafs*, and *ruh*—and connecting with God spiritually, through the *ruh*. It is often done sitting in any comfortable position, with eyes closed or open, and inner awareness and attention focused on the physical location of the heart while maintaining awareness of the entire body. A similar process or a word sometimes used in the same context is *tafakkur* (contemplation; Badri, 2000). The object of *tafakkur* is to contemplate on God, which can be done by focusing on God's creation or the inner spiritual center of the person. It is similar to the process of centering in the heart that I use as an intervention at the level of *qalb*, but the difference here is that rather than focusing on the emotional material or "black spots" on the heart in the process of discovering and uncovering the self, the focus here is on witnessing and connecting with God rather than the self. While I do not regularly use this intervention in therapy with all clients, I do often use it in cases of acute anxiety or panic attack, and with clients who are experiencing physical reactions as a result of trauma, as this practice can help a person cope with or sometimes even transcend the constriction of the bodily experience. I also introduce some forms of *muraqaba* or *tafakkur* with clients who are committed to following the outward practices of their spiritual path but are not finding that they are having any effect on softening their heart or increasing *taqwa*. In these cases, my aim with *muraqaba* or *tafakkur* is to try to get the clients to become aware of the *ruh* aspect of their self and to connect their actions with the intention of getting closer to God, through an internal awareness and opening to God's reality. The spirit is an important and integral part of the human being and when repressed or denied can have negative effects on the whole, resulting in imbalance and disease.

Ibadah. Within the Islamic paradigm, the primary mechanism for connecting directly with Allah is through *ibadah* (worship). In addition to religious acts of worship, *ibadah* includes anything that is done for the sake of God. It says in the Quran, "I did not create the *jinn* and mankind except to worship Me" (51:56). Great importance is placed on the preoccupation with *ibadah* because it is through these acts of devotion that people can come closer to God. They are the mechanisms by which we secure a direct line from our lower selves, mired in the separation of the *dunya*, to God's reality of *tawhid*, and the *ruh* is the part of our self that enables this link. Thus we can uncover our *ruh* and remain open to receiving God's love and guidance by keeping consistently engaged in *ibadah*.

In therapy with some of my Muslim clients, I recommend certain forms of *ibadah* in a variety of ways depending on the nature of the presenting problem and the client's relative spiritual orientation. In some cases, for those who do not pray or have stopped praying, for example, which is quite common, it is a matter of helping people reconnect or connect for the first time with spiritual practices as a source of balance and stability and helping them cognitively make the connection that doing these acts can positively affect and sometimes resolve the symptoms of which they are complaining. This is introduced as indicated by the client and adjusted to fit within his or her relative beliefs and the level of desired commitment to said beliefs.

Often I discover that although the person may be praying five times a day, for example, they are not praying with *khushu* (sincere intention in submission), and thus the act is reduced to a physical behavior without serving the purpose of connection to Allah. In some cases, if a person does not feel an established connection with God and feels alone or somehow forsaken, I suggest the practice of *dua* (supplication) as a way of opening a line of communication between the person and the divine source. I may make *dua* with clients in session, modeling the practice, asking God to open the client's awareness and witnessing of Him. In the

Quran, Allah says, "Call upon Me, I will answer" (40:60); Allah encourages developing a relationship of personal reliance on Him, through direct communication. I also do something similar even with people who do not believe in God by simply reorienting the terminology to be in line with their personal worldview. For example, I had a client who did not relate to the concept of God but did have a strong sense of a "spiritual force in the universe." While this intuitive sense existed in his psyche as a theory, he did not have a related practice that allowed him access to this perceived spiritual force. In my work with this client, I used the basic concept of *dua*, as a means of personal spiritual connection to something greater outside of the person, by helping the client attune to that force that he is aware of on his own terms, and to develop a relationship with it where he can access strength and reassurance.

While *dua* and other forms of *ibadah* are ways for us to communicate with God, within the Islamic paradigm the Quran is seen as a vehicle by which Allah communicates directly with us. In Islam, the Quran is the central source of guidance, where Muslims learn what Allah wants from them and find specific guidance to follow. However, in addition to receiving the relatively overt behavioral prescriptions from the book of Allah, it is believed that one can receive directly into the heart guidance from God through the recitation of the Quran. The Quran is considered a *shifaa* (healing) for humanity, meaning that not only is the knowledge in it a healing balm for our character to correct our actions and live in accordance with *fitrah*, it is believed that the actual words themselves can bring healing to our hearts in ways that transcend our limited intellectual capacity for understanding. Thus, simply reciting or listening to the Quran can bring *shifaa* to a person's heart and soul. Among other things, I use Quranic recitation as a treatment intervention with Muslim clients who have more severe mental illness, such as psychoses, where they have lost touch with reality. While often these clients need psychiatric treatment with medications and/or in residential treatment facilities, supplementing such treatment with Islamic psychotherapy can make significant advancements in treatment, especially with Muslim clients (Abdullah et al., 2013). Recitation of the Quran, among other forms of *ibadah*, often has the most success in grounding the person in the ultimate balance of metaphysical and temporal realities embodied in the Islamic paradigm.

Recommendations

While this approach is based on a theoretical orientation that is grounded in the Islamic tradition and has direct parallels with other practitioners operating from the same source material (for example, see Skinner, 2018, 2010; Keshavarzi & Haque, 2013), the development of a consensual model and overarching theoretical framework has yet to be formalized. Colleagues and I in this emerging field are actively involved in efforts toward this goal, but more development and support for such efforts are needed. For application of such models with Muslim clients, it is crucial that these efforts be grounded in Islamic knowledge, theologically sound, and validated by the global community of Muslim scholars (*ulama*).

Once that solid foundation is established, then we can build upon it to create further applications of such theory into practice. This effort should involve clinical research to provide a robust body of evidence to further substantiate the field of Islamic psychology as a legitimate body among the academic and scientific community that can position itself to offer significant contributions to humanity at large. Aspects of this framework and certain insights into the human psyche can be adapted to secular contexts while the framework as a whole can still maintain its Islamic integrity for applications within the Muslim community. This can then result in proper training and education programs for the development of more competent and well-informed practitioners to be operating from a standardized and approved model of Islamic psychotherapy for various populations. The potential for numerous applications across several fields is too vast to mention here, but suffice it to say this type of advancement could effect positive change on a wide scale.

For now, the exposure to and increased awareness of the work that is currently being done on a grassroots level by individual practitioners to serve the Muslim community and bring light to the insight into psychology that the Islamic tradition has to offer, as a result of efforts like this edited volume, will, *insha'allah* (God willing), be of good use to multiple audiences. For non-Muslim clinicians, my hope in presenting this approach to Islamic psychotherapy is to provide insight into some of the attributes of an Islamic paradigm of psychology that may be useful in considering their own approach to working with Muslim clients. It can be helpful to be aware of the sensitivities and particularities in working with believing Muslims, and some of the interventions that I outline in this chapter—*dhikr*, connecting with the ninety-nine names, the practice of *muhasabah*, for example—can be used as tools to help the client reach treatment goals. However, as with any recommendations in best practice, clinicians should work from within their relative level of expertise. As much of this Islamic approach is grounded in traditional knowledge that requires supervised instruction from qualified teachers, many of the interventions and techniques described here are not meant to be followed as a manual without proper training.

For Muslim clinicians, it is perhaps a matter of committing on a deep level to their own intimate knowledge and practice of the Islamic science of the soul and connecting it directly with notions of psychology, reorienting the Western paradigm while maintaining useful Western techniques, and adopting a new outlook and relationship to both psychology and Islam that embraces an indigenous Islamic paradigm. My hope would be not that potential practitioners would rely so much on these techniques as a manual that they deliver, but that they understand that of prime importance in this Islamic model of psychotherapy is the therapist's continual work on him- or herself. The model thus requires more that therapists be fellow humans on the path alongside clients who are experiencing and relating with them in the ongoing process of mastery of the human condition, rather than implementing a series of techniques at a distance from the client. The practitioners of Islamic psychotherapy must be relating and speaking from experience on the journey together with their clients.

In terms of gaining knowledge in this endeavor, a great many resources, although spread out in different subfields within the tradition, can be tapped into within the vast realm of Islamic knowledge of the soul. And for potential Muslim clients as well, my hope is that by gaining insight into the process of an Islamic model of therapy, the often present stigmas around counseling and mental health can be lifted. If understood in light of psychology, clients can potentially view the *deen* as a resource and a healing balm for most if not all of the struggles that people face daily. Perhaps most important of all, however, is that by outlining a practical approach to understanding and reforming the human soul with an Islamic theoretical orientation to psychology, we can inspire a wider audience of Muslims and non-Muslims alike to appreciate the insight that an Islamic psychological perspective has to offer in the knowledge of the soul (*ilm an nafs*).

References

Abdullah, C. H. B., Abidin, Z. B. Z., Hissan, W. S. M., Kechil, R., Razali, W. N., & Zin, M. Z. M. (2013). The effectiveness of Generalized Anxiety Disorder intervention through Islamic psychotherapy: The preliminary study. *Asian Social Science, 9*(13), 157–162.

Ashley-Farrand, T. (2008). *Healing mantras: Using sound affirmations for personal power, creativity, and healing.* Wellspring/Ballantine.

Awaad, R., & Ali, S. (2015). Obsessional disorders in al-Balkhi's 9th-century treatise: Sustenance of the body and soul. *Journal of Affective Disorders, 180,* 185–189. doi:10.1016/j.jad.2015.03.003

Awaad, R., & Ali, S. (2016). A modern conceptualization of phobia in al-Balkhi's 9th-century treatise: Sustenance of the body and soul. *Journal of Anxiety Disorders, 37,* 89–93. doi:10.1016/j.janxdis.2015.11.003

Badri, M. (2000). *Contemplation: An Islamic psychospiritual study.* Herndon, VA: International Institute of Islamic Thought.

Badri, M. (2013). *Translation and annotation of Abu Zayd al-Balkhi's sustenance of the soul.* Herndon, VA: International Institute of Islamic Thought.

Beck, A. T. (1976). *Cognitive therapy and the emotional disorders.* New York: International Universities Press.

Berne, E. (2010). *Games people play: The psychology of human relationships.* Penguin UK.

Breakwell, G. M. (1986). *Coping with threatened identities.* London: Methuen.

Compton, W. C. (2005). *Introduction to positive psychology.* Belmont, CA: Thomson Wadsworth.

Cuijpers, P., Sijbrandij, M., Koole, S., Huibers, M., Berking, M., & Andersson, G. (2014). Psychological treatment of generalized anxiety disorder: A meta-analysis. *Clinical Psychology Review, 34*(2), 130–140.

Dobson, K. S. (Ed.). (2009). *Handbook of cognitive-behavioral therapies*. New York: Guilford Press.

Duffy, K., & Veltri, D. (1998). *Interpreting in therapy: Getting out of the way. VIEWS*, 15(4). http://www2.palomar.edu/users/lmendoza/documents/Mental_Health_Interpreting.pdf

Ellis, A. (1962). *Reason and emotion in psychotherapy*. Secaucus, NJ: Lyle Stuart.

Ghazali, A. M. (1986). *Revival of religious learning* (F. Karim, Trans). New Delhi: Kitab Bhavan. (Original work published 1853.)

Hanh, T. N. (2016). *The miracle of mindfulness*. Boston: Beacon Press.

Hans, E., & Hiller, W. (2013). Effectiveness of and dropout from outpatient cognitive behavioral therapy for adult unipolar depression: A meta-analysis of nonrandomized effectiveness studies. *Journal of Consulting and Clinical Psychology, 81*(1), 75-88.

Haque, A. (1998). Psychology and religion: Their relationship and integration from an Islamic perspective. *American Journal of Islamic Social Sciences, 15*(4), 97-116.

Haque, A. (2004). Psychology from Islamic perspective: Contributions of early Muslim scholars and challenges to contemporary Muslim psychologists. *Journal of Religion & Health, 43*(4), 357–377.

Inayat, Q. (2005). The Islamic concept of the self. *Counselling Psychology Review, 20*(3), 2–10.

Jaspal, R., & Breakwell, G. M. (Eds.). (2014). *Identity process theory: Identity, social action, and social change*. Cambridge: Cambridge University Press.

Jerath, R., Edry, J. W., Barnes, V. A., & Jerath, V. (2006). Physiology of long pranayamic breathing: Neural respiratory elements may provide a mechanism that explains how slow deep breathing shifts the autonomic nervous system. *Medical Hypotheses, 67*(3), 566–571.

Jung, C. G. (1977). The face-to-face interview. In R. F. C. Hull's (ed.), *C. G. Jung speaking: Interviews and encounters* (pp. 424–439). Princeton, NJ: Bollingen Paperbacks.

Jung, C. G. (2013). *The psychology of the transference*. Abingdon, England: Routledge.

Keshavarzi, H., & Haque, A. (2013). Outlining a psychotherapy model for enhancing Muslim mental health within an Islamic context. *International Journal for the Psychology of Religion, 23*, 230–249.

Kettani, H. (2010, January). 2010 world Muslim population. In *Proceedings of the 8th Hawaii International Conference on Arts and Humanities* (pp. 12-16).

Kiev, A. (1964). Psychotherapeutic aspects of Pentecostal sects among West Indian immigrants to England. *British Journal of Sociology, 15*(2), 129–138.

Lings, M. M. (1995). *Muhammad: His life based on the earliest sources*. London: Unwin Paperbacks.

Lopez, S. J., Pedrotti, J. T., & Snyder, C. R. (2014). *Positive psychology: The scientific and practical explorations of human strengths*. Thousand Oaks: Sage.

Maqsood, R. W. (1995). *The Muslim marriage guide*. London: Quilliam.

McCullough, M. E., & Witvliet, C. V. (2002). The psychology of forgiveness. *Handbook of positive psychology*, 2, 446–455.

Moodley, R., & West, W. (Eds.). (2005). *Integrating traditional healing practices into counseling and psychotherapy* (Vol. 22). Thousand Oaks, CA: Sage.

Penedo, F. J., & Dahn, J. R. (2005). Exercise and well-being: A review of mental and physical health benefits associated with physical activity. *Current Opinion in Psychiatry*, 18(2), 189–193.

Reed, E. S. (1997). *From soul to mind: The emergence of psychology from Erasmus Darwin to William James*. New Haven, CT: Yale University Press.

Rogers, C. R. (1966). Client-centered therapy. Washington, DC: American Psychological Association.

Salmon, P. (2001). Effects of physical exercise on anxiety, depression, and sensitivity to stress: A unifying theory. *Clinical Psychology Review*, 21(1), 33–61.

Saraswati, S. S., & Hiti, J. K. (1996). *Asana pranayama mudra bandha*. Bihar, India: Bihar Yoga Bharati.

Schneider, K. J., Pierson, J. F., & Bugental, J. F. (Eds.). (2014). *The handbook of humanistic psychology: Theory, research, and practice*. Thousand Oaks, CA: Sage.

Seligman, M. E. (2004). *Authentic happiness: Using the new positive psychology to realize your potential for lasting fulfillment*. New York: Simon and Schuster.

Skinner, R. (2010). An Islamic approach to psychology and mental health. *Mental Health, Religion & Culture*, 13(6), 547–551.

Skinner, R. (2018). Traditions, paradigms and basic concepts in Islamic psychology. *Journal of Religion and Health*, 1-8. https://doi.org/10.1007/s10943-018-0595-1

Stewart, R. E., & Chambless, D. L. (2009). Cognitive-behavioral therapy for adult anxiety disorders in clinical practice: A meta-analysis of effectiveness studies. *Journal of Consulting and Clinical Psychology*, 77(4), 595-606.

Tajfel, H., & Turner, J. (1979). An integrative theory of intergroup conflict. In W. G. Austin & S. Worchel (Eds.), *The social psychology of intergroup relations* (pp. 33-47). Monterey, CA: Brooks/Cole.

Tajfel, H., & Turner, J. C. (1985). The social identity theory of intergroup behavior. In S. Worchel & W. G. Austin (Eds.), *Psychology of intergroup relations* (pp. 7–24). Chicago: Nelson-Hall.

Tan, S.-Y. (2003). Integrating spiritual direction into psychotherapy: Ethical issues and guidelines. *Journal of Psychology and Theology*, 31(1), 14–23.

Turner, J. C., Hogg, M. A., Oakes, P. J., Reicher, S. D., & Wetherell, M. S. (1987). *Rediscovering the social group: A self-categorization theory*. Oxford: Blackwell.

Utz, A. (2011). *Psychology from the Islamic perspective*. Riyadh, Saudi Arabia: International Islamic Publishing House.

CHAPTER 2

Utilization of Islamic Principles
in Marital Counseling

Layla Asamarai, PsyD

S o much of the literature available on working with Muslim populations emphasizes Muslims as a subgroup within a greater Islamic or Middle Eastern context. However, while there is growing information on preferred methods in working with them given their sociocultural framework (Dwairy, 2006; Sue & Sue, 2015; Daneshpour, 2017), far less common is information on how to work with this population from within their Islamic schemas and frameworks. This chapter aims to share information on working with Muslim clients with an emphasis on the use of Islam as a guide and tool, not only in rapport building but in effecting the process of psychotherapy.

It is ironic that I am contributing a chapter to this book, as I formerly was unable to see the necessity for Islamic psychology or any religion-based psychotherapy. I was among those who believed that good therapy was good therapy, and that it need not be religion based. I share my former stance because I, like many, was concerned that religion-based psychotherapy would pose a value infringement on individuals, and I was concerned that employing any religion-informed orientation might assume a religious dogma that would leave clients feeling judged or sanctioned. After working in Dubai with a predominantly multinational Muslim client base for over eight years, I found many clients to be defensive, distrustful, and uncomfortable with psychotherapy or counseling. In an effort to conscientiously provide culturally responsive services, I discovered that the need to bring forth Islamic principles was pressing, and failure to do so would risk estranging so many from partaking in counseling services. Many clients who identified as practicing Muslims considered psychology to be a Western practice and perceived it as a threat to the parts of Islam that they held dear, and this was at times also true of nonpracticing Muslims who still considered Islam to be the cornerstone for their families. I began seeking out potential bridges from within the Islamic tradition that were in agreement with a counseling framework and practiced bringing them forward. The fruit of this endeavor is what I share in this chapter.

Throughout this chapter, deidentified vignettes have been included to guide the discussion on how Islamic principles from the Quran and hadith were used to facilitate the process of marriage counseling. While this contribution alone cannot act as a doctrine on the use of Islamic marriage counseling, it is a brief thematic collection reflecting emerging experiential practice of Islamically informed marital counseling.

The Marital Union

The marital union is one of the most discussed topics in the Islamic tradition, both in the Quran and hadith. Marriage is not only a permissible act but one that is divinely decreed, blessed, and considered essential in completing an individual's religiosity. Prophet Mohammed (pbuh) was quoted as saying that "when one marries, half of faith is perfected" (Saheeh Al-Albani Saheeh al-Targheeb wa'l-Tarheeb, hadith 1916). Within Islamic Scripture, there is extensive discussion of the marital relationship, including but not limited to conflict, spousal selection, sexuality, communication, divorce, and even *how* to divorce. While Islam is considered a complete way of life for practicing Muslims, even for many nonpracticing Muslims it is very often considered the ultimate jurisdictional authority in matters of marriage and divorce. This information is supported by a recent Pew survey of Muslims in thirty-nine countries in which the majority of Muslims endorse Islamic Sharia law as governing their lives (Bell, 2013). It is not then surprising that when couples experience marital problems they are more likely to seek the assistance of an Imam or religious authority before considering a mental health professional (Aloud & Rathur, 2009).

Seeking Help

Mariam and Ahmed were newlyweds who arrived to the clinic together at Mariam's insistence. Frustrated with her feeling that her husband was "too attached" to his mother and not attentive enough to her, Mariam came to the clinic a week prior to learn how to "change him." When advised that the process of change is facilitated with both her and Ahmed working together, she agreed to come back to therapy, this time with him. As Mariam tearfully described how unhappy she had been feeling, Ahmed sat sheepishly on the edge of the sofa. Mariam continued to list all that she felt needed to change and in her frustration turned to Ahmed and said, "Say something!" Frustrated, Ahmed replied, "What do you want me to say?" and proceeded to state that her emotional outburst was unnecessary as she didn't need to see a psychologist to talk about such personal family matters. He went on to extend his disapproval to the study of psychology and how "a good Muslim relies only on Allah." "True believers," he announced, do not become mentally unwell, and if they did, it was a sign of distance from Allah.

This vignette highlights a number of important issues. First and perhaps most obvious is Mariam's desire to have sessions where she receives guidance on how to change Ahmed without him coming with her or even knowing about her plans. Second, not only did Ahmed refuse the idea of talking to others about his problems, he rejected the concept of mental illness and believed this to be opposed to being a "good Muslim."

Ahmed's perspective against seeking counseling is not uncommon in Muslim communities, where marriage counseling and other mental health services are still somewhat new and developing. Even when mental health services are sought, they are often accessed secretly. There remains a strong social stigma whereby seeking mental health services is considered shameful as it is perceived to be a lack of faith, weakness of character, and bad family upbringing (Aloud & Rathur, 2009; Amer, 2006; Erickson & Al-Timimi, 2001; Youssef & Deane, 2006). Further, even when problems do arise, seeking the help of a mental health professional was something only 11 percent of Muslims in midwestern America said they would do, while 21 percent said they would get help from a family member and 19 percent from a religious leader in the community (Aloud & Rathur, 2009). Mental health problems and marital problems are seen as a "private family matter" (Hamdan, 2009), and as such, any intervention that is seen as "other" is rejected.

Psychotherapy is a rather new intervention within Muslim communities. The idea that this treatment, born of Western ideology, could save one's marriage is considered by some as challenging the vitality and efficacy of Islam. As in the case of Ahmed and Mariam, there is often the harmful belief that someone who seeks mental health services has weak faith, as true believers cannot and should not succumb to adverse emotions. When it is difficult for clients to understand their emotionality, it is often important that therapists provide psychoeducation that normalizes the experience. Particularly in the case of practicing Muslims, receptivity to psychoeducation was higher when examples from the Islamic tradition were used. When working with Ahmed around understanding the sadness and grief he was experiencing, a hadith about when the Prophet Mohammed (pbuh) was seen weeping after the death of his infant child, Ibrahim, was shared with him. When asked by his companions how a messenger of Allah could cry, he responded, "Indeed the eye tears and the heart saddens" (Bukhari 23.62). Not only was the experiencing of sadness normalized by the Prophet, but so was crying in response to this grief. When the Prophet Mohammed (pbuh) himself admits to sadness and broken heartedness, how then can grief and depression be attributed to weakness of character or faith?

The utilization of hadith is powerful in laying the bedrock for counseling, yet still the question of how and why to treat an ailment with counseling (versus other spiritual or medical treatments) arises. While obtaining medical treatment for medical ailments is common practice in most Muslim communities, mental illnesses and psychosocial problems are not yet allotted the same understanding and permission. Meanwhile, this resistance to seeking mental health services is in direct opposition to Prophet Mohammed's explicit instructions to obtain treatment, namely his instruction to "heal your selves." He also said, "There is no ailment that Allah has created, except that He also has created its remedy" (Bukhari 7.582). Given the Islamic tradition of using Quranic recitation as a form of healing, introducing counseling as a "remedy" to clients is usually met with openness. Further, in laying out the therapeutic framework it has been helpful to utilize the Prophet's saying, "A believer is the mirror of a fellow believer" (Al-Adab Al-Mufrad 12.238). By sharing this hadith, clients are encouraged to contemplate on the reflective nature of a mirror as it gently reflects back what it is shown without harshness, command, or compulsion and to expand on how remedial it can be.

Speaking from within an Islamic interface was essential from the very beginning of working with this couple as I was only able to encourage Mariam to return with her husband upon reminding her of the Quranic verse that discusses the process of change. The Quran states that "indeed, Allah will not change the condition of a people until they change what is in themselves" (13:11). The awareness, desire, and motivation to change are prerequisite to God's change of a person, and for Mariam to attempt to circumvent this was contrary to Islamic teachings. Change was therefore not only a choice that Ahmed needed to make himself, it involved a conscientious process of which he needed to be a part.

Ahmed's insistence that Mariam should not have spoken with anyone about "family" affairs was a point of contention between them, but an opportunity to foster connection and understanding. Though it may be ideal that spouses directly address each other with their conflicts and complaints, to be allowed only this to the exclusion of any other resource is neither practical nor congruent with the Islamic position on the matter. The Quran states,

> And if you fear dissension between the two, send an arbitrator from his people and an arbitrator from her people. If they both desire reconciliation, Allah will cause it between them. Indeed, Allah is ever Knowing and Acquainted [with all things]. (4:35)

While it is often the case that a member from both her and his family are appointed with the task, many now seek treatment from Imams in local *masjids* who are seldom equipped to navigate the process of marriage counseling. Just as medicine has evolved from folk medicine administered at the hands of community elders, marital counseling is similarly an evolved format of a historically and religiously prescribed intervention. Interestingly, this verse inserts the condition that "if" a couple desires reconciliation, Allah will make it so. This verse places the responsibility to change or to intend to change first and foremost in the hands of the couple. This is essential because many Muslim clients possess fatalistic beliefs whereby they feel surrendered to fate and do not know how to command their voice and as such do not take responsibility for the choices made (Shah et al., 2008).

Ahmed and Mariam decided to keep coming for sessions, and eventually Ahmed called to book the appointments. Ahmed grew so interested in the process that he began to refer his friends and family and encouraged them to go to counseling in order to broaden their perspective on themselves and their lives.

Love and Intimacy

Lamya and Adel had been married for sixteen years and had four children. They arrived for counseling to avoid a divorce that they feared would hurt their children. The couple indicated that they shared a "sweet" engagement period, but that after marriage things turned sour. The bulk of their marital problems surrounded Lamya's complaints regarding Adel's long-standing disinterest in intimacy and sex, except to have children. In working with the couple, Adel shared that he could not think of Lamya in a sexual way and that he felt that to do so was to disrespect and dishonor her. Instead, Adel wrote romantic love poetry about Lamya, which he believed to be most honoring of her. Lamya harbored a lot of resentment about the numerous times she approached him in a desire to be intimate only to push her away and told to "fear God" and grow up. Adel defended his perspective by stating that sex was animalistic and that he was aiming for a higher, purer love with her.

Adel loved Lamya so much that his love for her inspired him to write nearly one hundred poems about his feelings for her, but Lamya could not feel his love in a way that resonated with her. The dissonance between what he felt and what she experienced was huge, and it needed to be addressed both conceptually and practically. Part of working with this couple involved Adel receiving some individual psychotherapy to address his negative beliefs about sex. In their work as a couple, it was vital that he begin to explore the universality and validity of his beliefs about love, sex, and marriage. Given that he reported himself to be a devout Muslim, it was through Islam that this process was initiated. It is stated in the Quran,

> And of His signs is that He created for you from yourselves mates that you may find tranquility in them; and He placed between you affection and mercy. Indeed in that are signs for a people who give thought. (30:21)

The verse brings no mention of love, and instead uses the word "affection." While love is mentioned in the Quran, it is never mentioned in discussing the marital union, and instead other words that provide more action-based qualities are mentioned. The presence of affection is far easier to jointly express and assess as a couple than the presence of love. Affection is an act, whereas love is a subjective feeling that Adel reported being overwhelmed with to the point of writing poetry, while Lamya felt unloved. When the Prophet was asked about his then deceased first wife, Khadijah, he indicated that he was "endowed [from God] with love for her" (Muslim 2435). This demonstrates how the presence of love is a divine offering that one can neither create nor destroy. In contrast, affection can be communicated in many different ways and involves the choice to be affectionate with one another. Although Adel reported the presence of a great love for Lamya, his relationship was struggling because he was not providing affection. The marital relationship is further described in the Quran, "They [spouses] are your garments and ye are their garments" (2:187), and in another verse it states, "It is He [God] who created you from one soul and created from it its mate that he might dwell in security with her" (7:189). Both of these verses illustrate a purposeful interdependence and togetherness between husband and wife.

From an Islamic perspective, sex is deemed not only permissible, but crucial and blessed when occurring within a lawful marital relationship

(Abd al Ati, 1977, p. 50). Further, there is overt mention of what kinds of practices are considered lawful as well as explicit instruction to engage in foreplay with specific mention of how foreplay is carried out (Khan, 2006). The following is an example of such clear mention of the nature of sexual relations between husband and wife:

> When one of you has sexual intercourse with his wife, he must always be conscious of her needs. If he finishes before her he then must not rush her and must wait for her until she is satisfied, because that frustrates her and prevents her from enjoying her sexuality.
>
> (Ibn Qudamah, as cited in Al-Hibri & El Habti, 2006, p. 211)

While marriage counseling helped Adel realize the magnitude of pain that Lamya had endured for such a long time, it also provided him an opportunity to safely explore his beliefs and assumptions. In his individual psychotherapy sessions it became evident that he had some maladaptive ideas about sex and sexuality and had held on to beliefs that sex was bad and dirty and that only dishonorable women could enjoy it. Adel had been unintentionally exposed to pornography at the age of ten and reacted with confusion and horror. Subsequently, when he told his father about it, he was punished and accused of "being bad." Adel became obsessed with trying to understand what he saw, which led to years of him secretly seeking out different kinds of pornography, and his first sexual experience was with a prostitute. Adel continued to struggle with his pornography addiction and felt immense shame. Upon working through his childhood experiences, he was able to draw parallels between his deeply ingrained beliefs that sex was bad, and could see the damage done to his relationship because of it. The transparency and openness fostered through their joint marriage counseling sessions proved to be additionally vital in helping him overcome the adverse childhood experiences that had been the source of his sexual problems. Adel was not only able to process his past and resolve it; he learned to foster and exchange affection with Lamya in a way that felt satisfying to each of them.

Responsibility and Power

Sara and Kareem were a newly engaged professional couple in their late twenties who were due to be married in less than six months but found themselves having a lot of disputes about finances. The couple, who identified themselves as progressive Muslims, met through friends after each rejected more traditional family-initiated arrangements. As they prepared for the wedding and marital life, Kareem suggested setting up a savings account that they could each contribute to monthly so that in a few years they could buy their own home. When Kareem began asking Sara about her salary to be able to complete the financial plan to buy a home, she grew very uncomfortable. Sara insisted that, in Islam, she had the full right to retain her wages (not contribute them to the household) and that household expenses were to be covered solely by Kareem. This seemed to be a side to Sara that Kareem had not anticipated, and since she earned 30 percent more than he did, he worried that he would be accused of financially exploiting her. At the same time, Kareem felt a great sense of injustice at the idea of working to support Sara while she collected her money. After his father left, Kareem was raised by his mother, who was the sole financial provider for the family. Moreover, he reported that he had never heard that Islam had such an arrangement. Sara, on the other hand, came from a home in which both parents were working professionals, but her father was the provider for the family and the mother's money was her own.

Sara's insistence that Kareem be the sole provider was based on the Quranic verse that states, "Men are in charge of women by [right of] what Allah has given one over the other and what they spend [for maintenance] from their wealth" (4:34). This verse places the responsibility of financial support solely on the husband, and from within this appointed responsibility, he is deemed in charge of the wife's welfare whether she has income or not. Due to the inheritance laws in Islam, some Muslim countries do not allow for joint banking, as there always needs to be a way to differentiate the husband's money from the wife's money. Discussions about finances and rights and responsibilities with Sara resulted in Kareem feeling that the relationship was more of a transaction and that he "worked for her." This conflict seemed to impose roles with which neither of them was fully comfortable. The couple was not aware of how they could be in adherence to Islamic principles and still come to an agreement that worked for them.

Couples like Sara and Kareem find themselves caught between Islamic tradition and present-day values, where men and women share power and finances. While it is a woman's right to receive full financial support from her husband without having to contribute any of her own finances, there is no prohibition in Islam against her contributing to the family wealth. One of the questions I posed is whether a wife's increase in financial contribution would result in power sharing or a proportional increase in power since the husband's position in the marriage is based on his financial responsibility. Upon reading about their rights and responsibilities, many couples like Sara and Kareem don't know if they are allowed to choose another way of organizing their relationship, and many couples are seeking Islamic clergy that are more progressive and willing to depart from misogynistic practices that are commonly misattributed to Islam. Prophet Mohammed's first marriage to Khadijah is a great example of a nontraditional marital arrangement that is starkly different from what many Muslims think to be the Islamic way. Not only was the Prophet twenty years younger than she, Khadijah was a businesswoman for whom he worked, and upon admiring his honesty and integrity, she proposed to him in marriage. Khadijah's wealth remained hers after marriage as was consistent with Islamic guidelines, though when the Prophet was boycotted, she spent from her wealth to support him and his companions (Taqra, 2015).

The marital union in Islam is both sacred and contractual (Abd al Ati, 1977, p. 57). The implications of this, especially in countries where the legal system is based on Sharia law, indicate that unless a fatwa (jurisprudential ruling) is obtained on a given matter, a default would be applied in the case of death or divorce. Kareem and Sara sought out various Islamic scholars to discuss their dilemma with them and created a premarital agreement whereby it was agreed that Sara would be a "partner" and would contribute 15 percent of her salary and that she would own a percentage of assets commensurate with her contributions.

While Sara and Kareem worked together to figure out an amicable arrangement, it was also important for them that their relationship did not become so transactional that they lost sight of the sacramental bond between them. The Prophet's life with Khadijah, his most beloved wife with whom he had a monogamous marriage for twenty-five years (Taqra, 2015), represents the balance between duty and kindness and demonstrates an equivalence between husband and wife rather than tit-for-tat equality. This distinction is made in the Quran, where it is stated, "Women shall have rights similar to the rights upon them; according to what is equitable and just" (2:228). Awareness and accessibility to these resources are essential for practicing Muslim couples in the process of negotiating their relationships as well as their identities and roles within those relationships. To be able to honestly and gently discuss these topics and share impressions and listen to the other is vital in being able to grow as a couple while discussing money, power, and responsibility. The Prophet said, "Whenever gentleness is added to something, it adorns it; and whenever it is withdrawn from something, it leaves it defective" (Riyadh Al-Saliheen 1.635). When the Prophet's wife Aisha was asked how he spent his time when he was at home, she replied, "He would do chores for his family" (Al-Adab Al-Mufrad 30.538). Prophet Mohammed was a gentle man who led by example and said, "The best of you is the one who is best to his spouse, and I am the best of you to mine" (Sunan Ibin Majah 3.9.1977).

Loyalty and Infidelity

In this section, I share two vignettes to highlight these themes.

Vignette 1

Reem and Hamad were married for over twenty-five years and had raised six children together. They came to counseling after Reem learned that Hamad had taken a second wife. Although they had married out of love, he had taken a new wife who was over a decade younger than Reem. Reem added that Hamad's new wife, whom he met at work, was newly pregnant and that this enraged her, especially since her youngest child with Hamad was fifteen years old. Hamad rested his head on his hand and sighed as Reem sobbed. Hamad expressed confusion with how badly she reacted and announced that he didn't do anything unlawful and that this was his religious right. Reem shared that many of her friends upon speaking with her told her that she needed to be patient because this (taking another wife) was his right and that he didn't do anything unlawful, but she emphasized that she didn't care because a "betrayal is a betrayal" and he was unfaithful. Hamad was upset by this statement and indicated that any good wife should love her husband enough to care whether he disobeys God or not. Hamad stated that he loved her very much and that he was being fair between Reem and his other wife. He described how he was evenly allocating his time and money between both wives. In the course of counseling, Reem disclosed that her father had taken another wife when she was eight years old and subsequently deserted them, and that she never thought that Hamad would be "that kind of a man" and then announced that she had wasted her love on and her years with him.

There are differences of opinion in Islam about polygamy and when and how it can be carried out. Without entering into that debate in this chapter or in sessions with clients, it is vital to make one major acknowledgment: even though polygamy may be lawful, it can still hurt. Though polygamy cannot be deemed a form of infidelity, as it is considered an acceptable practice in Islam, it is normal for the wife to feel betrayed. The lawfulness of this practice often takes away the support that women need, leaving them to suffer in silence and shame. They are scolded for their unholy reaction, which adds insult to injury. As a result of this social estrangement, women often say that it would be better if the husband had an unlawful affair than marry someone. Even Prophet Mohammed acknowledged the pain it causes a woman when he prohibited his son-in-law Ali from taking another wife while married to his daughter Fatima, indicating that it would hurt Fatima and what hurts Fatima would hurt him (Sahih al-Bukhari 67.163).

While the lawfulness of polygamy may be debatable in many Muslim circles, this discussion is misplaced in sessions with clients like Hamad.

Hamad not only believes himself to be doing something lawful but considers himself to be honorable as he is committing to a marital relationship (rather than an affair) where he is responsible and accountable. He considers himself unjustly attacked when he has gone to great lengths to avail his finances and resources to be responsible for both wives without reducing Reem's quality of life. Hamad saw himself as distinctly different from her father, who abandoned his family after taking another wife, and felt unappreciated by her insinuation that they were the same.

After the birth of their son, Hamad's second marriage ended in divorce due to irreconcilable differences. Reem remained married to Hamad, and even though he divorced his second wife, Reem was neither able to reconcile things nor was she able to trust him not to do it again. Her relationship with Hamad became platonic, and she indicated that she remained with him only for the children's sake. Reem refused to do any work on her childhood experiences with her father and said that she didn't want to think about any of those things and would devote her life to her children. Reem was afraid to "open the wounds of the past." Her decision to devote her life to her children was tainted with hopelessness and despair that she was attempting to anesthetize through selfless dedication to her children and a magical wish that she would just forget. Working through her childhood or current relationship was frightening for her, as all she could see waiting were more pain and hopelessness. As Reem's children grow into adulthood, it is possible that she might begin to question her own well-being and seek counseling again. However, at the conclusion of therapy, she made the decision to focus her attention on the role of motherhood, as she thought it would help her feel more productive and successful than that of her role as a wife.

VIGNETTE 2

Amal and Sameer were a married couple with one child. They came to therapy per Sameer's insistence after repeated arguments in which Amal insisted that he was cheating on her. Sameer repeatedly swore to Amal that he was faithful and that he would never be with another because he loved her and to commit adultery would be a major sin in Islam. No matter what Sameer said, he could not convince Amal. While initially confused by her accusations, over time he grew less sympathetic and became increasingly irritated and offended. Amal could not explain why she was so suspicious of him and would become very upset. With the permission of her husband, Amal asked to meet with me alone. In her individual session, she shared that while they were engaged, she had cheated on Sameer with a former fiancé and she was now sure that he would do the same to her. She expressed immense remorse for what she had done and was afraid of losing Sameer to another woman but felt destined to lose him because of what she had done. In exploring her insistence that he would cheat on her, she said that it was a well-known fact that "adultery is a debt" and "whomsoever cheats will be cheated on." She could not cite the origin of these sayings except to say that they were common knowledge and that maybe they were Islamic.

Amal's guilt was not unique to her and is normal; however, her ideas about how she was destined to be cheated on were destroying the very relationship she was so afraid to lose. It was vital to explore the validity of these two beliefs and to also compare them to Islamic principles. The Quran clearly states, "Each soul is responsible for its own actions, no soul will bear the burden of another" (6:164). Further, adultery is considered a major sin in Islam, and for Sameer to have to endure such a transgression against his soul just because Amal did so would be unfair to him. While laying out an accurate theological position on the matter was beneficial, it was vital that the couple also examine the underlying psychological causes behind their conflict. Amal, who was always a daddy's girl, knew that her father had female friends on the side. Despite this knowledge, she resented and blamed her mother for his actions. Amal detested her mother's weakness and "stupidity" for not discovering her husband's cheating and for not being good enough so that her father wouldn't cheat. In Amal's therapy, she worked through various childhood experiences, one of which was being her father's keeper and helping her to see how damaging it was to be entrusted with such information. Amal wept when she realized that, since childhood, she had thought that she was "bad" and had been shouldering responsibility for her father's choices. Amal worked not only on self-forgiveness but also on releasing herself from the responsibility of her parents' marriage, as well as the guilt of having a marriage better than theirs.

Reconciliation

Fatima and Khalil were married for twenty years and had five children. They sought counseling because Fatima insisted on getting a divorce. She indicated that she had "had enough" and that she didn't love Khalil anymore. Fatima wept as she talked about how Khalil had taken another wife fifteen years earlier and how she endured and was patient for the sake of her children. Khalil was adamant that Fatima was "not in her right mind" and even thought that she was possessed by a demon and had recently taken her to a sheikh to remove the possession, but to no avail. Fatima grew very angry as he shared all that he had done to save his marriage. She was adamant that she wanted a divorce and would not accept any form of reconciliation. Fatima and Khalil both wanted peace, but he wanted it through reconciliation and she through divorce. Khalil was disappointed when he realized that the counseling sessions would not serve the purpose of convincing her to reconcile and stay in the marriage. Similarly, Fatima was frustrated at the invitation to openly and respectfully dialogue with Khalil about what she wanted and expressed suspicion that these strategies were ploys to get her to back down from the idea of divorce. It was crucial to clarify the goals of marriage counseling as well as the role of the therapist.

Khalil and Fatima were both full of fear. He was afraid of losing a twenty-year marriage and having to deal with the implications that come with such a divorce for their family. Meanwhile, she was afraid of losing her choice and being forced to remain unhappy because that is what had been deemed best for the children. It was important to be able to bring something from within Islam to help ameliorate the situation and also to bring a few things into perspective—namely, even God does not infringe on an individual's free will. He states in the Quran, "There shall be no compulsion in religion" (2:256). If God, the creator, does not force anyone to worship Him, how is it that we humans can be so comfortable forcing individuals to do what they do not want to do? Further, Islam does not forbid divorce and allows both the husband and wife to end the marital union (Abd al Ati, 1977, p. 220). Fatima wanted so badly for Khalil to agree to the divorce because she wanted to make sure that he would not harm her with child support or spousal support and worried that he would take out his anger about the divorce on their children. While Khalil denied that he would ever do such a thing, he refused to cooperate with her desire to obtain a divorce. By the time they arrived in my office, they had been at war with each other for a year and a half, exhausting them and their families After validating Khalil's desire to hold on to his family and fear of things falling apart, I reminded him of what is stated in the Quran for husbands to "either retain with righteousness, or release with benevolence" (2:229). Two months later, while sitting together in her family's home, he cried as he agreed to divorce her, and in subsequently narrating in my office the events of that day, she also cried. Despite the battles between them, eventually he did release her with benevolence, and she felt it. It is stated that "if they both desire reconciliation, Allah will cause it between them" (4:35). This verse poses an important question regarding what reconciliation can mean; while it may mean for the couple to heal their conflicts and continue together, other times it may be a merciful resolution of the issues through a benevolent parting of ways.

Conclusion

Islam is so often described by practicing Muslims as a way of life. Even for nonpracticing Muslims, it is often considered a culture of practices that often represents fairness and due process. The provision of Islamically guided marital counseling proved powerful in each of the cases presented. To set aside Islamic praxis would in many instances steer clients from a source of trust and truth and subsequently risk estranging them from psychological services. As was presented in these vignettes, some outcomes were more favorable than others, but in each case the infusion of Islamic principles helped clients engage more completely and confidently in the process. Because this Islamic infusion was implemented more by need than by a purposeful Islamic theoretical orientation, it was essential to do a lot of background reading and studying on verses from the Quran and various chapters of hadith that could be used to buttress Western psychotherapeutic theories or practices. In researching various sources, it is essential to discern the partiality of one's own degree of religious observance and how liberal or conservative one is as one explores the vast array of religious interpretations. Further, it is critical that providers attempt to be as impartial as possible and to invite clients to discuss discrepancies in interpretation among sources and scholars while disclosing one's own biases.

In addition to using Islamic-friendly terminology and an Islamic theoretical framework for therapy, there is also a pressing need to address ideas that can be seen as un-Islamic within psychotherapy. One major concept that meets with a lot of resistance seems to emerge when it becomes necessary to address a client's childhood or family of origin. Islam holds parents in very high standing, right after God, as evidenced by the verse that says, "And your Lord has decreed that you not worship except Him, and to parents, good treatment. Whether one or both of them reach old age [while] with you, say not to them [so much as], 'uff,' and do not repel them but speak to them a noble word" (17:23). Herein exists a deep conflict in individuals needing to address adverse experiences involving their parents in their histories but who fear committing blasphemy. In working with clients who have struggled with whether they are "bad" to discuss wrongs involving their parents, it has proven essential to talk about how therapy is a practice aimed at healing rather than exposing the pains of the past. While there is often a lot of resistance to talking about painful experiences from childhood, particularly that might make parents "look bad," it has been helpful to discuss the Prophet's childhood, which was full of adversity and pain, and to highlight his example of openly talking about his childhood. Some clients also express a lot of guilt about backbiting loved ones or family in session, as this behavior is prohibited in Islam. They are often unaware that when one is sharing the information for the sake of seeking help, it is permissible (Riyad-us-Saaliheen 256). Further, because most clients would agree that their parents did not intend to cause harm, healing the resulting hurt is one of the best ways to free themselves of the pain and move beyond the past into more authentic and honoring relationships with them. This perspective has been met with great relief as clients intentionally and mindfully heal themselves in order to heal their relationships and begin to see that as a form of honoring their parents.

While this chapter portrays a number of instances where Islam was utilized in a clinical setting, it remains that the applications described were organic attempts born out of culturally responsive care that led to the weaving of Islamic principles into an existing integrated cocktail of Western psychotherapy, rather than the intentional establishment of an Islamic theoretical framework. Islamic psychology remains in its infancy but holds great potential given the high attunement to the self, the mind, and the heart in Islamic tradition and teachings. The development of an Islamic psychology theoretical framework holds great promise in the conceptualization of diagnosis and treatment. Not only would treatments be compliant with the Islamic tradition, they could serve to reinforce and heal from within the Islamic way of life that many observant Muslims adopt.

References

Abd al Ati, H. (1977). *The family structure in Islam*. American Trust Publications.

Al-Hibri, A., & El Habti, R. (2006). Islam. In D. S. Browning, M. C. Green, & J. Witte (Eds.). *Sex, marriage, and family in world religions*. (pp. 150–225). New York: Columbia University Press.

Aloud, N., & Rathur, A. (2009). Factors affecting attitudes toward seeking and using formal mental health and psychological services among Arab Muslim populations. *Journal of Muslim Mental Health, 4*, 79–103. doi:10.1080/15564900802487675

Amer, M. M. (2006). *When multicultural worlds collide: Breaking down barriers to service use*. Paper presented at the annual meeting of the American Psychological Association, New Orleans.

Bell, J. (2013). *The world's Muslims: Religion, politics, and society*. Washington, DC: Pew Forum on Religion and Public Life.

Daneshpour, M. (2017). Family therapy with Muslims. New York: Routledge.

Dwairy, M. A. (2006). Counseling and psychotherapy with Arabs and Muslims: A culturally sensitive approach. New York: Teachers College Press.

Erickson, C. D., & Al-Timimi, N. R. (2001). Providing mental health services to Arab

Americans: Recommendations and considerations. *Cultural Diversity and Ethnic Minority Psychology, 7*, 308–327. http://dx.doi.org/10.1037/1099-9809.7.4.308

Hamdan, A. (2009). Mental health needs of Arab women. *Health Care for Women International, 30*, 595–613. http://dx.doi.org/10.1080/07399330902928808.

Khan, M. A. (2006). *Sex & sexuality in Islam.* Lahore, Pakistan: Nashriyat.

Shah, S. M., Ayash, C., Pharaon, N. A., & Gany, F. M. (2008). Arab American immigrants in New York: Health care and cancer knowledge, attitudes, and beliefs. *Journal of Immigrant and Minority Health, 10*, 429–436. http://dx.doi.org/10.1007/s10903-007-9106-2.

Sue, D. & Sue, D. W. (2015). *Counseling the culturally diverse: Theory and practice.* New York: Wiley.

Taqra, M. (2015). *The tale of Lady Khadijah Bint Khuwaylid, wife of Prophet Muhammad SAW.* [Kindle DX version].

Youssef, J., & Deane, F. P. (2006). Factors influencing mental-health help-seeking in Arabic-speaking communities in Sydney, Australia. *Mental Health, Religion & Culture, 9*(1), 43–66. doi:10.1080/13674670512331335686

The HEART Method: Healthy Emotions Anchored in RasoolAllah's Teachings

Cognitive Therapy Using Prophet Mohammed as a Psycho-Spiritual Exemplar

Farah Lodi, MA, CCC

> There is a beautiful role model in the Messenger of God for those
> of you who have set their hopes on God and the hereafter and
> always remember God abundantly.
>
> (Quran 33:21)

THIS CHAPTER is written from the perspective of a Muslim Western-educated cognitive behavior therapist. I practice in an integrative way using an Islamic spiritual approach when appropriate. Being an American Muslim, born in Africa of South Asian descent, has enabled a heightened sense of multicultural sensitivity that is integral to my work. A decade ago I moved to Dubai, where I teach psychology at Zayed University, and also own a small counseling practice where I see a wide range of ethnically diverse clients with anxiety, depression, and phase-of-life and relationship issues.

A client's initial assessment and diagnosis start with an intake form that includes a question about religious identity. For many of my Muslim clients, Islamic values are deeply ingrained in their lifestyle, so they ask to incorporate these in their therapy. I do this primarily by disclosing my own spiritual identity as a Muslim, when needed, in a subtle, genuine, and respectful way, without in any way imposing my beliefs upon the client. In the same natural way, I help the clients express their personal spirituality. This not only facilitates a deeper client/therapist bond based on a shared belief system, but, also brings consciousness of Divine Reality into the room, which can be powerful and transformational. Clients have reported that this realization manifests as a positive energy that motivates them to actively participate in the session as they are cognitively reminded that they are part of a meaningful Divine plan. For me, this energy translates into compassion for my clients as I inwardly pray for their beneficence and actively seek to help them in the most considered, consistent, and effective way.

My case conceptualization relies on the belief that each person's soul comes from God and returns to Him. This is echoed in the Muslim prayer "From God we come and to God we return." The soul originates from the breath of God (38:72), and since we all come from the same Divine source, we are bound together in unity, reflecting the Islamic principle of *tawheed* (oneness). For me, this absolute truth facilitates unconditional positive regard for my clients. Since the soul comes from the Divine, it seeks contentment through closeness to God, but this spiritual instinct can be suppressed by the desires of the *nafs*, which is a powerful internal pull toward self-centeredness and worldly pleasures. My therapeutic orientation is based on the belief that the teachings of Prophet Mohammed help us control the *nafs*. When the client can relate to this understanding of life, then my treatment plan combines cognitive behavioral therapy (CBT) with what I call the HEART Method: Healthy Emotions Anchored in RasoolAllah's Teachings. This is a foundation for counseling based on spiritual modeling of RasoolAllah (also known as Prophet Mohammed or the Messenger of God).

Islamic psychology emphasizes thoughts affecting emotions. This is clearly alluded to in the Quran:

> Whoever believes and acts aright, they shall have no fear, nor
> shall they grieve.   *(6:48)*

This verse acknowledges what I like about CBT. I understand it to mean that a core belief in God and His Messenger, in conjunction with abiding by the code of conduct outlined in the Quran, facilitates resiliency. In CBT terms, this verse is saying that our thoughts influence our core beliefs, and when these are aligned with purposeful actions, a healthy meaning in life is present, promoting psychological well-being. Therefore, CBT is very Islam-friendly, and Islam is infused with CBT. I integrate CBT and the HEART Method by using tools such as psycho-education, cognitive restructuring, behavior activation and behavior experiments, mood tracking, and spiritual modeling. When the intake form and initial interview clarify that the client can relate positively to Prophet Mohammed as a spiritual exemplar, then I help the client use this belief as a resource to facilitate his or her own resiliency. At the end of the day, the process of change is what it's all about. I help the client track progress at regular intervals by using clinical measurement tools such as the Becks Depression Inventory and self-report scales to check reduction in self-harm behaviors and improvements in subjective well-being. A client feedback form is used at regular intervals to make sure that therapy goals and expectations are being met. When setting and tracking these goals, we keep in mind the Quranic verse,

> God will not change the condition of a people until they change what is in themselves. (13:11)

Although each case is different, a HEART Method counseling session may begin with acknowledging the Divine presence. This can be done simply by beginning with the affirmation "I begin with God's Name, the Most Merciful, Most Kind." To introduce the Prophet as an exemplar in the early stages of therapy, we may discuss Quranic verses such as,

> O you who believe, pay heed unto God and His Messenger, and do not turn away from Him now that you hear His message. (8:20)

As mentioned earlier, this helps set the stage, and for some clients it shifts them from feeling overwhelmed and helpless to feeling spiritually supported. In order to understand why I embrace a methodology steeped in the *sunnah* (practices of Prophet Mohammed), we must first understand the significance of RasoolAllah for Muslims.

Prophet Mohammad: A Spiritual Exemplar

Prophet Mohammed (570–632), also known as RasoolAllah, is the single most studied and documented figure in history, with an extensive literature review available, making him a most relevant clinical research subject. Muslims believe that he is the last Prophet and Messenger of God. This reverence is embodied in the *Shahada*, which is one of the five pillars of Islam that all Muslims are supposed to profess: "There is no God but Allah, and Mohammed is His Messenger." RasoolAllah is an exemplary figure to be emulated as it is believed that he was spiritually pure and a perfect human with Divinely inspired knowledge and therefore unique cognitive frames.

The word "Islam" means to surrender, and Muslims believe that the central meaning and purpose in life are to surrender to God. Muslims believe that the *sunnah* constitute the perfect illustration of surrender to God (Armstrong, 2006). They also believe that when there are mental or emotional health issues, then the spirit needs treatment and attention, just like the physical body does during illness (Ghazali & Yusuf, 2010). Those who view everything the Prophet Mohammed did as infinitely meaningful and relevant believe that there is a potent transformational aspect to his example. This chapter provides the theoretical background and conceptual framework for the HEART Method. The paradigm is derived mainly from a psychological analysis of the Prophet's behaviors as well as related quotes from the Quran.

A study of his life shows that RasoolAllah had a multidimensional, psycho-spiritual approach to coping with negative life events. This can be broken down into specific steadfast and predictable teachings from his life that are core components to the HEART Method. These teachings are as follows:

- *Taqwa* and *tawakul*: he had a deeply ingrained schema of *taqwa* (God-consciousness) and *tawakul* (reliance on and trust in God).
- Compassion: he had a compassion-based schema that included sincere goodwill toward all of creation.
- Acknowledging and accepting challenging emotions: he was attuned to his emotions.

- ► Reframing: he reframed thoughts so as to be aligned with a belief in the hereafter.
- ► Talking to God: he spoke to God through *dua* (direct communication), *salah* (ritual prayer), and meditation (contemplation).
- ► Quranic code of conduct: he followed the laws outlined in the Quran, which promote prosocial behaviors.

These teachings constitute the HEART Method. Prophet Mohammed said, "There is an organ in the body, that if it is pure, the whole body is pure, and if it is diseased, the whole body is diseased—the heart" (Bukhari). This echoes the CBT principle that adaptive thinking leads to positive emotions and actions, while maladaptive thinking can lead to negative emotions and actions. Many Muslim clients find it useful to associate therapy with the essentially vital heart, an organ believed to be the center of consciousness (Ghazali & Yusuf, 2010). CBT identifies the brain as a command center, but in my work with Muslims, we also focus on the heart, which emanates love of God and the Prophet, as the source for inspiration and resiliency.

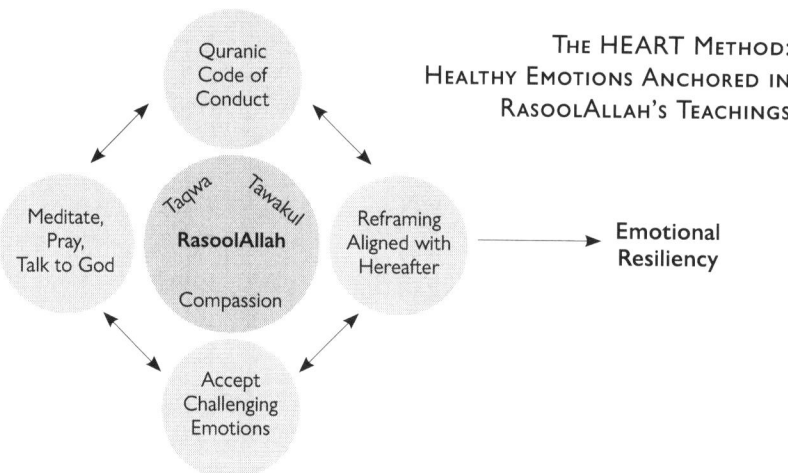

THE HEART METHOD: HEALTHY EMOTIONS ANCHORED IN RASOOLALLAH'S TEACHINGS

A study of the *seerah* (biography of Prophet Mohammed) shows the teachings of the HEART Method to literally be at the heart of the Prophet's emotion-regulation system, hence this apt title. In this chapter, I discuss how the Prophet emulated these teachings, together with empirical evidence that validates them as scientifically sound, and I describe how in counseling sessions I integrate RasoolAllah's teachings with CBT.

Taqwa and Tawakul-Based Schema

Over the course of his life, Prophet Mohammed faced a full range of psychological stressors, such as grief and loss, rejection and abandonment, humiliation, war, betrayal, poverty, and migration—but he didn't succumb to anxiety or depression because he actualized an "inner life," characterized by the Islamic concepts of *taqwa* (God consciousness) and *tawakul* (reliance on God). According to Islamic tradition as seen in the writings of Ghazali and Ibn Arabi, these spiritual virtues provide an orienting belief system that brings a Muslim closer to God and therefore to a state of happiness (Ghazali & Yusuf, 2010). The Prophet's example is to nurture these inner spiritual dimensions, which are ultimately both cognitive schemas and coping mechanisms, and they can be explained to the client as such through the narration of numerous stories.

Perhaps the best narrative from the Prophet's life that showcases all the teachings of the HEART Method is the incident of abuse that he experienced in the city of Taif. This event is a good point of reference for psychological analysis. The Prophet referred to it as the most difficult day of his life, and it occurred in what is known as the "year of sadness," when he lost his beloved wife and uncle who raised him, and the Muslim community was on the verge of starvation due to economic sanctions. Historical accounts describe how the Prophet went to Taif for help, but was attacked, insulted, and cast out (Lings, 1983). The Quran says that God gave RasoolAllah the option of destroying his enemies, but he chose to forgive and pray for them instead. In his well-documented prayer at Taif (which I refer to throughout this chapter), the Prophet exemplified resiliency:

O Allah, I complain to You of my weakness, my scarcity of resources and the humiliation I have been subjected to by the people. Oh, Most Merciful of those who are Merciful! Oh Lord of the weak and my Lord too! To whom have You entrusted me? To a distant person who receives me with hostility? Or to an enemy to whom you have granted authority over my affair? So long as You are not angry with me, I do not care. Your favor is of a more expansive relief to me. I seek refuge in the light of Your Face by which all darkness is dispelled and every affair of this world and the next is set right, lest Your anger or displeasure descends upon me. I desire Your pleasure and satisfaction until You are pleased. There is no power and no might except by You.   (*Lings, 1983, pp. 88–89*)

Here, RasoolAllah had absolute awareness and reliance on God, spoke to God, acknowledged challenging emotions, reframed the situation in line with the bigger picture, and engaged in prosocial behaviors of compassion and forgiveness, thereby staying optimistic; this buffered him from feelings of despair. This story of Taif encapsulates the HEART Method and can be used with clients to demonstrate how the method works.

Another example of the Prophet's *taqwa* and *tawakul* can be seen in the incident at the Cave Thawr. He and his companion Abu Bakr were being pursued by enemies who wanted to kill the Prophet. In order to seek protection, they hid in the cave of Thawr for three days. At one point the enemies came so close to the entrance of the cave that Abu Bakr could see them above him. Fearing for the life of the Prophet, he whispered, "Messenger of God, if they look down toward their feet they will see us!" The Prophet replied, "Abu Bakr, how can you fear for two men whose constant companion is God himself?" (Haykal, 1976). The Quran states, "Then God sent down His *sakînah* [calmness, tranquility, peace] upon him, and strengthened him with forces that you saw not" (9:40).

Taqwa doesn't have a single meaning, but can be understood holistically. It has been described as an all-encompassing inner consciousness to obey God and stay away from what is forbidden (Bhatti et al., 2015). In his theory on spiritual intelligence, Hussain (2014) says that *taqwa* "expresses a state of alertness, awareness and attentiveness, and a meticulous sense of duty to God" (p. 17). Therefore, *taqwa* is a moral and ethical source for actions. Growing empirical evidence links *taqwa* to resiliency. Rosmarin et al. (2013) measured the relationship between belief in God (similar to awareness of God) and treatment outcomes for psychiatric patients. Results showed that a higher belief in God corresponded with greater improvements in psychiatric well-being, suggesting that an internalized belief in God is psychologically protective.

Tawakul is defined as trust in, or reliance on, God. If *taqwa* is a cognitive state of Divine awareness that attributes everything to Divine will, then *tawakul* may be its emotional counterpart, translating into a feeling of trust in God and reassurance of His mercy. According to Bonab and Koohsar (2011), *tawakul* is a lens that allows a Muslim to be aware of God in everything and everywhere. Krause and Hayward (2015) defined *tawakul* as the confident belief that God is taking care of one's best interests. Empirical studies show the significance of *tawakul* in the reduction of anxiety and depression. According to Pargament's et al. (1990) study, religious beliefs are often utilized as coping mechanisms, with the most common religious coping mechanism cited in numerous studies being trust in God. In the discussion, Pargament et al. (1990) describe trust in God as belief in a just, loving, and omnipotent God; trust in His will; emotional reassurance from an intimate relationship with Him; positive framing of problems; and an external locus of control that helps individuals accept their own limits (p. 802). Although the study focused on Christian participants, all the above values may be generalized to Muslims as these are common beliefs to all monotheistic religions.

Taqwa and *tawakul* can be seen as analogous to a recognized psychological construct: God as a secure attachment figure. Both Ghazali in the eleventh century and Bowlby in the twentieth theorized that secure attachment leads to psychological resiliency. Ghazali & Yusuf (2010) said that to achieve happiness we need to have a positive relationship with and be close to God. Bowlby (1907–1990) defined certain attributes relevant to an attachment figure, such as availability during distress and responsiveness in times of need, which can apply to a Muslim's relationship with God, as mentioned in the Quran:

> So, put your trust in God and rely on Him alone if you are
> indeed believers. (5:23)

> Put your trust in God, He suffices as a Guardian.
>
> (33:3)

> For individuals who rely on God, God will prove all sufficient.
>
> (65:3)

In both examples of Taif and the Cave Thawr, the Prophet exemplified submission and absolute certitude in God, resulting in optimism. Therefore, it is reasonable to reevaluate *taqwa* and *tawakul* as not just spiritual coping mechanisms and cognitive schemas, but evidence-based psychological constructs linked to resiliency.

A HEART Method session would include an explanation of these concepts and how the Prophet practiced them, combined with the supporting scientific evidence that can motivate Muslim clients to increase their *taqwa* and *tawakul*. RasoolAllah was optimistic in any situation, often saying that "truly Allah is with us." To help clients feel closer to God, they can be asked to contemplate upon the wonders of creation. Chapter 55 of the Quran (Surat al-Rahman) offers a poetic description of cosmic reality that is *taqwa*-inspiring. A useful exercise to help clients who ruminate is to use all five senses to savor blessings: look at five beautiful colors, listen for four sounds, touch three nice objects, smell two fragrances, taste one good thing. This simple cognitive technique is known as "grounding," which interrupts obsessive thinking. When *taqwa* and *tawakul* are practiced repeatedly, cognitive distortions such as "disqualifying the positive" are replaced with an awareness that good things are all around us, too. Another intervention is to encourage the client to consciously stick to a positive view of God's plan. This can be done by reading supporting verses from the Quran, such as the following:

He is with Us wherever we are.   (57:4)

To Allah belongs the east and the west; wherever you go, there
is the Face of Allah.   (2:15)

This helps the client step back from a problem and look at it with a balanced view that includes many possibilities rather than the catastrophic
view with which many anxious or depressed clients initially present.

To work on *tawakul*, the client could be asked to recognize that if
something is not happening, it's God's will and not indicative of personal
failure. This can reduce feelings of helplessness, especially for those with
perfectionist and obsessive compulsive disorder (OCD) tendencies.
Numerous verses in the Quran can be discussed and given as homework for reflection:

Allah is Omnipresent, Omniscient.   (2:115)

Whoever has mindfulness of Allah, Allah grants a way out
and provides for them in ways they could never imagine.
                                                            (65:2–3)

Some common automatic negative thoughts can be challenged in the
following way:
  ► "I'm a failure": Allah says the believers are successful (23:1).
  ► "No one can help me": It's upon Us to help the believers (30:47).
  ► "I'm too sinful": Allah loves those who repent (2:222).
  ► "Life is too hard": He wants ease for you (2:185).
  ► "I can't cope": Allah will not burden a soul with more than it can
    bear (2:286).
  ► "I'm unappreciated": Your efforts and striving will be appreciated
    (76:22).
  ► "I'm worthless": We have indeed honored the children of Adam
    (17:70).
  ► "I'm alone": He is closer to us than our jugular vein (50:16).

> "I want more in this life": The hereafter is better and more enduring (87:17).

Quranic verses can be laminated and used as affirmations and coping cards, or they can be silently recited with contemplation. A *taqwa/tawakul*–based tool that many of my Muslim clients use is *istakhara*, or seeking Divine guidance through a special prescribed prayer. The belief is that through *istakhara* the best path opens up automatically. This can help a client accept an outcome, even if this wasn't their desired outcome, since it's attributed to Divine will. A concept that I help clients understand is that the opposite of "depressed" is not "happy," but rather "acceptance." Acceptance based on the Islamic belief system that everything that happens is ultimately good for us can reduce anxiety.

Compassionate Schema

RasoolAllah was an extraordinary exemplar of compassion, advocating it as the basis for all relationships, even when distressed. As mentioned earlier, at Taif, the Prophet forgave and prayed for his abusers. This compassionate schema, even while he was under threat, helped him avoid vengeance or retaliation and instead to focus on problem solving.

Another example of the Prophet's compassion is when, after being persecuted and banished from Mecca for many years, he later reentered the city as a conqueror, saying to his former enemies, "I say to you as Joseph said to his brothers: no blame upon you today. Allah will forgive you, and He is the Most Merciful of the Merciful" (Quran 12:92).

In effect, the Prophet forgave many who had tried to torture, persecute, and kill him. A compassionate stance helped him deal with his enemies with empathy, avoiding conflict and establishing good relationships. When people approached RasoolAllah with uncomfortable topics such as fornication or adultery, he listened to them with respect and helped them. The Prophet said that the best of people are those with the most compassion, who aid creation the most. There was an incident when the Prophet reached for his head covering but a cat had fallen asleep upon the cloth; to avoid disturbing the cat, RasoolAllah carefully cut a small piece of the fabric from one edge, enough to cover his head.

In another example, the Prophet's adversarial neighbor would throw garbage in front of his house every day to provoke and taunt him. One day she did not perform this hostile ritual due to an illness, so the Prophet went to visit her out of concern for her well-being. She was so impressed with his character that she consequently became Muslim. Many times he assertively stood his ground, such as when he negotiated political alliances, so RasoolAllah was steadfast when needed.

A great deal of research has been done on the link between compassion and psychological resiliency. Based on an analysis of fifty-five peer-reviewed studies, Oman (2011) said that compassion is consistently recognized as an important positive psychological factor, and he cited numerous empirical findings that link compassion to enhanced self-esteem, positive mood, better relationships, and better health. Paul Gilbert (2010), founder of compassion-based CBT, defines compassion as "behavior that aims to nurture, look after, teach, guide, mentor, soothe, protect, and offer feelings of acceptance and belonging in order to benefit another person" (p. 217). He theorizes that humans process and balance all emotions through three internal emotional regulation systems: we can be in a state of "threat" when we perceive danger to our well-being, in a state of "drive" when geared toward achievement, or in a state of "soothing" when content (Gilbert, 2010). A resilient person fluctuates adaptively between these states depending upon the situation; the critical element for successfully navigating from one emotion to another is compassion. So, to shift from feeling threatened to feeling soothed (without getting stuck in aggression, for example), or to change from feeling excessively driven to feeling content (without arrogance, for example), an individual needs a compassionate mindset. RasoolAllah had a compassion-based schema that enabled him to navigate through these three emotional systems in a way that kept him calm and positive.

In HEART Method sessions, stories of Prophetic compassion and the associated psychological benefits can be discussed. Therapists can ask clients, "How would a compassionate mindset affect you?" To help clients actualize compassion, I use role play and the Gestalt empty-chair technique, combined with questions such as "What do you think it must be like to be in the other person's shoes?" Compassion-based interventions in couples' therapy are especially effective, where partners are encouraged to do small acts of kindness for each other daily and to think compassionately rather than critically about each other. This increases the positivity factor in the relationship, which, according to marriage therapist Dr. John Gottman, leads to couples turning toward rather than away from each other—a key factor for marital success.

As Gilbert theorizes, self-compassion is critical for resiliency. Muslim clients can appreciate a spiritual rationale for self-compassion as they think about the Islamic belief that God breathed His Spirit into Adam (38:72). Acknowledging this Divine spark that we all contain can form the basis for self-worth, self-esteem, and building self-efficacy. The story about a prostitute who was forgiven because she gave water to a thirsty cat (Hadith Muslim) can help the client realize that there are no limits to God's mercy, and just like God forgives us, so must we forgive ourselves in order to move forward. These ideas can help clients who self-loathe or self-harm.

Accepting/Acknowledging Challenging Emotions

Prophet Mohammed's trust in God helped him to lay bare his feelings. In his oft-cited prayer at Taif, RasoolAllah talked about his emotions: "O Allah, To Thee I complain of my weakness, my lack of resources and my lowliness before men." This is a clear acknowledgment of vulnerability. In another example, when the Prophet buried his sixth child, Ibrahim, he cried publicly. When questioned by his companions regarding this show of emotion, he said, "I have not commanded against sadness, but against raising one's voice in lamentation. What you see in me is the effect of love and compassion in my heart for my lost one" (Haykal, 1976).

According to CBT philosophy, emotions arise from how we think. It's important to be aware of and process emotions; if suppressed they can lead to physical problems such as pain and inflammation, and overwhelming emotions can lead to maladaptive coping strategies such as substance abuse and addictions. Most psychotherapeutic interventions revolve around understanding and accepting negative emotions, which is the first step to releasing and processing them. Shalcross et al. (2010) cite several studies that link acceptance of emotions to reduced symptoms of panic, decreased rumination, better emotional regulation, and better stress tolerance.

In her widely acclaimed work on emotion-focused therapy for couples, Sue Johnson advocates the importance of facing vulnerable emotions in order to have healthy relationships (*Hold Me Tight*, 2009). Her research shows that when one partner is able to express his or her feelings to the other, it releases bottled-up emotions and usually elicits empathy, thus promoting open communication, better problem solving, and higher levels of satisfaction in the relationship.

In a HEART Method session, I remind clients that at Taif the Prophet spoke to God from the heart, explicitly mentioning feelings of weakness and humiliation. Early in the counseling process, clients may have difficulty talking about emotions such as remorse and shame. One way to help them open up is an adaptation of the game Jenga, where a tower of wooden blocks has to be dismantled one block at a time without letting the tower fall. Each block has a different emotion-related word written on the bottom, such as "guilt," so as the clients remove that block, they have to describe what guilt means to them and a time when they felt guilty. These are icebreakers that work well with teenagers and young adults, helping to desensitize them to being emotionally vulnerable. I often remind self-conscious clients that RasoolAllah cried, too, and that tears are a natural way of releasing the stress hormone cortisol.

Another helpful intervention is for clients to write a "healing letter," in which they address a range of challenging emotions, starting sentences with "I feel hurt when. . . . I feel angry when. . . . I feel humiliated when. . . ." This can help them express how they really feel, leading to an emotional release and acceptance of a difficult situation.

Reframing

Reframing involves challenging negative thoughts and beliefs and replacing them with thoughts aligned with truths. Muslims believe that the Prophet ascended to the heavens and met God during the event known as Isra Al-Miraj, so it is believed that he saw Divine Reality firsthand, which gave him the natural ability to reframe everything according to the bigger picture. RasoolAllah viewed this life as preparation for the much more important hereafter; he taught Muslims that how they perform in this world would determine their state in the next world, so for Muslims, all cognitive interpretations should function around this reality.

An example of prophetic reframing is when a man came to Prophet Mohammed confessing he had committed sins with a woman to whom he was not married. The Prophet emphasized that something bad can turn into something good as he recited this Quranic verse: "And establish prayer at the two ends of the day and at the approach of the night. Indeed, good deeds do away with misdeeds. That is a reminder for those who remember" (11:114). One of his sayings summing up his ability to reframe is:

> Wondrous is the affair of the believer for there is good for him in every matter and this is not the case with anyone except the believer. If he is happy, then he thanks Allah and thus there is good for him. If he is harmed, then he shows patience and thus there is good for him.
>
> *(Muslim 2999)*

In their study, Pearce et al. (2015) developed religiously integrated CBT treatment plans for depression. Muslim patients were taught to reframe their thinking by using the Quran and Islamic practices in order to form healthy thinking. The findings were that the patients who received religiously integrated CBT treatments showed greater improvement than those treated with other psychotherapies (Pierce et al., 2015).

In a HEART Method session, reframing can be taught in a practical way. CBT thought records can be filled out with the help of HEART questions, similar to Socratic questions, to challenge negative thinking:
- What does the Quran teach me about this?
- When I think of how the Prophet handled Taif, can I handle my problem differently?
- What spiritual practice that helped me in the past can help me now?

- How important is this problem really, if I look at the bigger picture?
- How am I affecting others? Is my behavior aligned with the Quranic code?
- How does my behavior affect my hereafter?
- What would RasoolAllah do?

The resulting new ideas can shift a client from automatic negative thoughts to more realistic and adaptive thinking. The thought record exercise helps clients acknowledge the CBT principle that thoughts are just thoughts; they can cause confusion and are not necessarily true. Through reframing, clients can be encouraged to understand their role and place in the universe in relation to the bigger picture. For example, a client who is stuck in depression due to infertility can be encouraged to reframe in accordance with the Quran's repetitive reminder to look after orphans, which may give the client a renewed meaning in life. Also useful are affirmations that reframe the situation in line with the temporary nature of all problems, such as the very hope-inspiring Quranic verse,

> With every difficulty there is ease, with every difficulty there is ease. (94:5–6)

For Muslims, pain and suffering can be reframed as a potential way of achieving reward in the hereafter since, according to the Quran, every atom's weight of difficulty will be rewarded in the hereafter:

> And the weighing on that day will be definite. So those whose scales are heavy, they are the successful. (7:8)

Helpful, too, are verses that recognize a Higher Power that is actually in charge:

> You may dislike something although it is good for you, or like something although it is bad for you. God knows and you do not. (2:216)

This keeps a practical focus on the reality that the problem will pass and is not in a person's control. It also frees the client from the burden of absolute self-reliance. All the above Quranic verses can be presented as coping cards and can be included in the mechanism of CBT thought records.

Talking to God / Prayer / Meditation

Talking to God is direct personal communication with the Divine. This can be done in different ways, including talking from the heart (*dua*), ritual prayer (*salat*), and meditation (contemplation). As Armstrong (2006) says, the Prophet had a higher state of consciousness, attuned with Divine Reality. At Taif, RasoolAllah exemplified the practice of talking to God from the heart when he said: "O, Allah, to thee I complain of. . . . I seek refuge in the light of Your Face."

Hussain (2014) says that prayer is a "sincere call, an earnest appeal and a humble request" (p. 58). In their review of Poloma and Pendleton's prayer scales, Black, Pössel et al. (2014) cite studies showing that prayer is positively associated with well-being and negatively associated with anxiety. In another study Oman and Bormann (2015) discuss the effects of mantra repetition (repetition throughout the day of a short spiritual phrase, to interrupt rumination). Results showed improved mental health, higher life satisfaction ratings, and reduction in depression and anger.

An abundance of peer-reviewed literature is available on the positive effects of mindfulness meditation on mental health. Oman et al. (2009) studied the effects of Easwaran's Eight Point Program (EPP). The EPP is recognized as a social cognitive meditation program with cross-cultural validity that consists of "empirically successful and conceptually generative strategies, usable within any major spiritual or religious tradition" (Oman et al., 2009, p. 21). The study concludes that the eight meditation practices, which closely resemble Prophet Mohammed's meditative habits, result in enhanced compassion, altruism, empathy, forgiveness, and self-efficacy. These eight practices are as follows:

1. Passage meditation: The Prophet spent many hours meditating upon Quranic verses.

2. Repetition of a holy word: The Prophet engaged in *zikr*, which is focused meditation upon and repetition of holy words, such as the ninety-nine Divine names of God. Repeatedly focusing on a word linked to patience, forgiveness, compassion, or gratitude supports retention of its meaning and integration of it into behavior (Oman & Borman, 2015).

3. Slowing down: The Prophet set priorities and spent time on inner reflection.

4. Focused attention: He spent much time in seclusion in the Cave Hira, meditating with deep concentration.

5. Training the senses: He filtered everything according to *taqwa*, *tawakul*, and compassion.

6. Putting others first: He taught that humans are God's vice-regents on earth, responsible for selfless goals.

7. Spiritual association: He encouraged people to spend time with others on a spiritual path.

8. Inspirational reading: The first words of the Quranic revelation are, "Read, in the name of your Lord." Seeking knowledge is a core value taught by the Prophet.

In a HEART Method session, clients should never feel judged on their religious practice, and there should be no pressure to impose any of the rituals of the five pillars. Even though these are significant, we have to meet clients where they are. Without underestimating the value of *salat* (ritual prayer), clients can be encouraged to think of prayer in different ways and to practice what helps them. Those who are emotionally overwhelmed can be encouraged to simply talk to God in a focused and heartfelt way. The client can be reminded of this verse:

> Wake up your certainty in Allah before you call upon Him in your dua. You will feel Him close to you more than the extent of your voice or even the vibrations of your larynx.
>
> (2:186)

I usually recommend to clients that they spend a few minutes each day in a quiet, comfortable spot. I encourage them to start with a sincere intention, to breathe slowly and deeply, and to clear their mind and talk to God—to really seek Him. When done properly (mindfully), there can be a transformational cognitive shift toward an enlightened awareness of Divine support. Similarly, in order to be beneficial, *salat* should be done with focused attention and a comprehension of the memorized verses; these both illuminate the prayers. When clients absorb the message of *surat al-Fatiha* (the first chapter of the Quran), which is repeated several times during *salat*, the references to praise, thanks, God's majesty, mercy, and the straight path have the potential to form new and possibly more optimistic neural pathways. Whatever way it's done, talking to God involves *taqwa* and *tawakul*. The relationship with God and RasoolAllah is alive and dynamic, so clients often feel changed in some way from it. They can be reminded of this powerful verse:

Call on Me and I will answer you. (40:60)

When appropriate I use a three-minute guided meditation technique, with repetition of "There is no God but God" combined with slow deep breathing, muscle relaxation, and mental visualization. While still in a state of meditation, the client can reflect and see lessons in life. Clients measure their pulse before and after this meditation; usually the pulse comes down, demonstrating a reduction of cortisol and increase of serotonin. They are also asked to track their mood before and after and usually report feeling "lighter." Meditation can thus be used as a CBT behavior experiment. However, some clients with post traumatic stress disorder (PTSD) may not respond well to meditation as it can trigger traumatic memories. Similarly, meditation can activate a spike in pain for clients with chronic pain, so this needs to be assessed beforehand using information from medical reports and the intake form.

Prosocial Behaviors from the Quran

Prophet Mohammed taught that humans are vice-regents on earth as well as servants of God—so they need to behave in ways that promote good relationships with God, nature, and others. In essence, this is a blueprint for living in harmony with creation. Armstrong (2006) says that the Quran gave the Prophet a mission "to create a just and decent society in which all members are treated with respect" (p. 13). Prophet Mohammed was truthful, honest, just, sincere, patient, grateful, and God-conscious (Bhatti et al., 2015). He did not mention people's faults and did not involve himself in that which didn't concern him. He held a good opinion of others, and he interacted with others with the best of manners, even when their behavior was unbecoming. RasoolAllah personally experienced oppression, violence, and discrimination, but his life is replete with acts of personal forgiveness, patience, gratitude, humility, tolerance, and many other prosocial behaviors. The Quranic code of behavior modeled by Prophet Mohammed provides skills for tolerating problems and developing adaptive coping strategies to deal with stressful events. The following are some examples of how prosocial behaviors enhanced his resiliency.

Forgiveness

The story of Taif is a classic example of forgiving his enemies. In another example, the Prophet forgave Hind (the wife of Abu Sufyan), who brutally mutilated the body of his beloved uncle Hamza. He was following a code of conduct explicit in the Quran:

> Keep to forgiveness Oh Mohammed, and enjoin kindness,
> and turn away from the ignorant. (7:199)

Forgiveness is a response to interpersonal conflict that involves the regulation of negative emotions and represents a prosocial and compassionate alternative to avoidance and revenge (Sandage & Jankowski, 2010). In their study on the relationship between forgiveness and resiliency, Worthington and Scherer (2004) concluded that forgiveness robustly predicts resiliency.

Patience

RasoolAllah was in an active state of patience, always holding firm to what would please God. This can be seen in his lifelong relationship with his beloved uncle Abu Talib, who was a father figure. It is unclear whether Abu Talib accepted Islam on his deathbed, but he did not accept Islam during his life, which was a source of frustration and personal anguish for the Prophet. However, he treated this family relationship with care and remained patient, compassionate, and close to his uncle, despite fundamental differences in beliefs. Prophet Mohammed's *taqwa* allowed him to patiently accept that if his uncle did not convert to Islam, then that was God's will. The Prophet's relationship with Abu Sufyan (the leader of the Quraish tribe) is characterized by many years of rivalry, where Abu Sufyan led military campaigns against him, opposing and relentlessly oppressing him and his followers. The Prophet handled this relationship with patience, taking the higher ground and forgiving Abu Sufyan for all past transgressions when he accepted Islam. The Quran says,

> O ye who believe! Seek help with patient perseverance and prayer: for Allah is with those who patiently persevere.
>
> (2:153)

> Give good tidings to the patient, who when disaster strikes them they say: indeed, we belong to Allah and indeed to him we will return. Those are the ones upon whom are blessings from their Lord and mercy.　　(2:155–57)

In *The Empath's Survival Guide* (2017), Orloff describes patience as "a coping skill, a spiritual practice, the practice of waiting, watching and knowing when to act" (p. 9). It is a calm and centered response to frustration, and a precursor to doing the right thing. Numerous peer-reviewed studies link patience to the ability to tolerate distress and to more positive affect.

GRATITUDE

RasoolAllah's attitude toward gratitude can be summed up in one example. His wife Ayesha recounted how he would stay up all night praying until his feet swelled up, and when she questioned him as to why he, who had no sins, was praying all night, he replied, "Should I not prove myself to be a thankful servant?"

> Show thy gratitude to Allah. Any who is grateful does so to the profit of his own soul. (31:12)

Gratitude is widely recognized as an important predictor of well-being, with hundreds of studies supporting the correlation of gratitude with enhanced resiliency.

In a HEART Method session, attention can be focused on RasoolAllah's personal vigilance; he was always conscious of how he dealt with others. There are certain key attitudes, based on the ethical and moral behaviors that RasoolAllah modeled, that clients can adopt to help change the dynamics of challenging relationships.

- ► **RasoolAllah looked at others with a positive view.** Clients can be reminded that when you see good in someone, then you are more likely to be content with them. Clients can be asked to make a list of a difficult person's good qualities. This can motivate the client to keep the peace with that person, be sensitive to the other's needs, not say things that hurt, and not judge. They can think about their own mistakes with that person and how to rectify them by seeking or giving forgiveness and consider how to avoid making the same mistakes by changing the situation that facilitates them.
- ► **RasoolAllah wanted good for others.** This was his state of heart (he even prayed for the abusers at Taif). Clients can be asked to subtly help a difficult person and note how altruism makes them feel. They can be asked to pray for that person and track their own mood before, during, and after these selfless acts.
- ► **RasoolAllah veiled others' shortcomings.** He taught us to turn a

blind eye, not to point out faults. This reduces gossiping and back-biting, which are a cause for breaking down relationships. Clients can be reminded that not everything should be tackled head-on and that it's useful to ignore certain things, to use humor, or to let it go.

CBT is based on the principle that if you change yourself, then negative patterns can change. To make this realistically manageable, clients can be asked to pick one prophetically inspired behavior change each week and make it part of their lifestyle. They can track how this change affects them, and once it's habituated, they can pick another behavior to work on. To motivate them throughout therapy, they can be reminded of these Quranic verses:

> There has come to you from Allah a light and clear book. By which Allah guides those who pursue His pleasure to the ways of peace and brings them out from darkness into light, by His permission, and guides them to a straight path.
>
> (5:15–16)

> The Holy Quran guides to the straightest way. (17:9)

Conclusion

The teachings of the HEART Method are not new; indeed, they are commonsense principles that were taught by all the prophets. But due to current geopolitical trends, Islam is not commonly associated with these teachings, and we have lost touch with the spirit of RasoolAllah's message, which is based on love and compassion. The HEART Method is anchored in a transformational relationship with RasoolAllah—a relationship unlike any other. It uses inspiring behaviors modeled by RasoolAllah combined with compelling cognitive reinforcements mainly derived from the Quran to create new emotional experiences for the client. The goal of the HEART Method is to help the client develop resiliency through the belief system associated with love for the Prophet.

The HEART Method needs to be presented as gentle reminders

of the Prophetic example, not as hard-core prescriptions. Obviously there are many variances within Islam, but the exalted spiritual rank of RasoolAllah is acknowledged by all Muslims, and the teachings showcased here are taken from indisputable primary sources. At times, differences in theological interpretation occur, so when this happens, it should be handled with the graciousness that the Prophet exemplified. He always made people feel respected by giving them his full attention, and he attracted people to Islam with his perfect manners. So as a therapist I, too, must give my full attention and be flexible with dogma. Not all six teachings have to be advocated. Meeting the client's needs may require just one Prophetic example for a breakthrough. Joining with the client is key. This means integrating and applying what makes the client happy. For example, when the client embraces pop culture, then lyrics like "shake it off" (Taylor Swift) and "I need to take it easy, easy, easy" (Drake) work as excellent emotionally uplifting affirmations, together with

God does not burden a soul with more than it can bear.

(2:286)

Challenges to the HEART Method can occur when clients are so overwhelmed that they are unable to stabilize catastrophic thinking. This can happen when there is severe trauma, active substance use, or a personality disorder. Also difficult is when clients come to therapy with rigid, uncompromising, or intolerant views that are incompatible with a compassionate mindset. CBT with the HEART Method may not be the preferred treatment in these cases.

Moving forward, clinical results from the HEART Method need to be examined empirically. This treatment plan should be manualized so it's available as a tool for therapists and as a self-help resource. A mobile app, with structured steps for utilizing Prophetic-based interventions, can be developed. Also, this plan could possibly be used as preventative care at college counseling offices and promoted as a psychological wellness campaign at the public health level in communities. The HEART

Method has clinical utility because it provides treatment that is not just generally Islamically oriented but specifically based on the spiritual modeling of RasoolAllah, providing a new, practical, and evidence-based dimension to the limited psychological therapies that are available for Muslims.

Combining CBT with the HEART Method has helped my clients develop psychological hardiness, as measured in quantifiable post-termination follow-up surveys. Many clients have reported feeling a comforting calmness and peacefulness in the counseling room when RasoolAllah is discussed. I attribute this to their cognitive shift toward hopefulness and an increase in serotonin levels as their soul responds to an innate attraction to the Divine. This is exhilarating for me, consequently enriching my professional competency. On a more personal level, it has strengthened my own relationship with Prophet Mohammed in an indescribable way. Finally, the HEART Method strategies can also be adapted to suit non-Muslim clients. When analyzed in depth, Prophet Mohammed's positive thinking, healthy behaviors, and remarkable psychological resiliency make him stand out as a universally appealing, excellent human being. RasoolAllah is a "mercy to the universe" (21:107) and therefore an exemplar for *all* of creation. May peace and blessings be upon him.

References

Armstrong, K. (2006). *Muhammad.* San Francisco: Harper Collins.

Bhatti, O. K., Alkahtani, A., Hassan, A., & Sulaiman, M. (2015). The relationship between Islamic piety (taqwa) and workplace deviance with organizational justice as a moderator. *International Journal of Business and Management, 10*(4), 136–153.

Black, S. W., Pössel, P., Jeppsen, B. D., Tariq, A., & Rosmarin, D. H. (2014). Poloma and Pendleton's (1989) Prayer Types Scale in Christian, Jewish, and Muslim praying adults: One scale or a family of scales. *Psychology of Religion and Spirituality, 7*(3), 205–216.

Bonab, B. G., & Koohsar, A. A. H. (2011). Reliance on God as a core construct of Islamic psychology. *Procedia-Social and Behavioral Sciences, 30*, 216–220.

Ghazali, A., & Yusuf, H. (2010). The m*Marvels of the Heart: Science of the Spirit. Ihya Ulum Al-Din—The Revival of the Religious Sciences.* Louisville: Fons Vitae.

Gilbert, P. (2010). *The Compassionate Mind.* Oakland: New Harbinger Publications.

Haykal, M. (1976). *The Life of Muhammad.* Petaling Jaya: American Trust Publications.

Hussain, M. (2014). *7 steps to spiritual intelligence: Based on classical Islamic teachings.* Markfield, UK: Kube Publishing.

Krause, N., & Hayward, R. D. (2015). Assessing whether trust in God offsets the effects of financial strain on health and well-being. *International Journal for the Psychology of Religion, 25*(4), 307–322.

Lings, M. (1983). *Muhammad: His life based on the earliest sources.* London: Islamic Texts Society.

Oman, D. (2011). Compassionate love: Accomplishments and challenges in an emerging scientific/spiritual research field. *Mental Health, Religion & Culture, 14*(9), 945–981.

Oman, D., & Bormann, J. E. (2015). Mantra repetition fosters self-efficacy in veterans for managing PTSD: A randomized trial. *Psychology of Religion and Spirituality, 7*(1), 34–45.

Oman, D., Thoresen, C. E., Park, C. L., Shaver, P. R., Hood, R. W., & Plante, T. G. (2009). How does one become spiritual? The spiritual modeling inventory of life environments (SMILE). *Mental Health, Religion and Culture, 12*(5), 427–456.

Orloff, J. (2017). *The empath's survival guide: Life strategies for sensitive people.* Boulder, CO: Sounds True.

Pargament, K. I., Ensing, D. S., Falgout, K., Olsen, H., Reilly, B., Van Haitsma, K., & Warren, R. (1990). God help me (I): Religious coping efforts as predictors of the outcomes to significant negative life events. *American Journal of Community Psychology, 18*(6), 793–824.

Pearce, M. J., Koenig, H. G., Robins, C. J., Nelson, B., Shaw, S. F., Cohen, H. J., & King, M. B. (2015). Religiously integrated cognitive behavioral therapy: A new method of treatment for major depression in patients with chronic medical illness. *Psychotherapy, 52*(1), 56–66.

Rosmarin, D. H., Bigda-Peyton, J. S., Kertz, S. J., Smith, N., Rauch, S. L., & Björgvinsson, T. (2013). A test of faith in God and treatment: The relationship of belief in God to psychiatric treatment outcomes. *Journal of Affective Disorders, 146*(3), 441–446.

Sandage, S. J., & Jankowski, P. J. (2010). Forgiveness, spiritual instability, mental health symptoms, and well-being: Mediator effects of differentiation of self. *Psychology of Religion and Spirituality, 2*(3), 168–180.

Shallcross, A. J., Troy, A. S., Boland, M., & Mauss, I. B. (2010). Let it be: Accepting negative emotional experiences predicts decreased negative affect and depressive symptoms. *Behavior Research and Therapy, 48*(9), 921–929.

Worthington, E. L., & Scherer, M. (2004). Forgiveness is an emotion-focused coping strategy that can reduce health risks and promote health resilience: Theory, review, and hypotheses. *Psychology & Health, 19*(3), 385–405.

CHAPTER 4

Conducting Spiritually Integrated Family Therapy with Muslim Clients Utilizing a Culturally Responsive Paradigm

Afshana Haque, PhD, LMFT-S

FOR MANY MUSLIMS, their Islamic values can be a great source of healing and comfort. A Muslim's faith and spirituality can provide meaning and illuminate dark times of hopelessness. Nevertheless, mental health professionals (MHPs) must practice caution in assuming that Muslims are monolithic in their experiences of faith and spirituality. Like all people who affiliate with religious denominations, Muslims vary in their levels of faith, spirituality, and religiosity. Elements of the culturally responsive paradigm as well as the philosophical underpinnings of collaborative language systems (CLS) can help MHPs navigate the therapy process when working with Muslim clients from a variety of religious experiences.

Culturally Responsive Family Therapy

Family therapists value a systemic approach in the assessment and treatment of a client. A systemic perspective requires understanding an individual's intrapsychic workings within the context of her relational, familial, and social environments. Culturally responsive therapy (CRT) assumes it is not possible for an individual to have experiences outside the influence of one's social environment, which includes socioeconomic status, ethnic and cultural background, historical context, minority status, and so on (Seponski, Bermudez, & Lewis, 2013). Many of these factors can enhance or diminish the therapeutic process; therefore, not only is it imperative to work within these contexts but also to address issues around poverty, language barriers, structural racism, segregation, social isolation, and distrust toward institutions (Seponski et al., 2013). Furthermore, consideration of the client's traditions, worldviews, and community support systems will expand the possibility for positive therapeutic outcomes and strong therapeutic alliance with the MHP.

The CRT approach also advocates for the use of cultural consultants, such as community members or religious leaders, not only to assist with the therapeutic process but also to ensure that the professional is not inflicting further oppression or marginalization (Seponski et al., 2013). Having cultural consultants can alleviate the fears of Muslim clients who worry that their values will be compromised if they see a non-Muslim MHP. Muslim MHPs should also be keenly aware of their own social location and how it differs from their Muslim clients so as not to either overidentify or assume that the clients' values align with their own.

For some Muslims, especially those from collectivistic cultures, the therapy process is largely misunderstood and highly stigmatized. On many occasions, I had college students with limited income request therapy sessions and who were worried about their parents finding out. In these circumstances, I would explain that people above the age of eighteen are legally considered adults; therefore, their parents are not obligated to sign any paperwork. So it would be up to the clients whether they wished to inform their parents about their involvement in therapy. Without the knowledge and support of their parents, student clients could only afford to pay lower rates. A culturally responsive therapist should be prepared to make such accommodations as well as respect and validate such fears.

Working with marginalized populations requires consciously creating an environment that is amenable to the client. The therapeutic alliance begins even before the first session. A free twenty-minute initial consultation helps clients feel more at ease regarding the therapy process, having already spoken to the therapist at least once. It also gives the therapist an opportunity to answer and explain the therapy process and the limits of her services, if needed, instead of wasting valuable session time. Providing a sliding-fee-scale option, scheduling around prayer times, and being mindful of Muslims needing to break fast during the month of Ramadan may also increase accessibility to therapy. Since Muslim therapists and other MHPs who market themselves as culturally responsive are fewer in number, having the option for online therapy through HIPAA-compliant videoconferencing software provides more options for the Muslim client.

The Muslim Context

Muslims reside in countries all over the world, and the practice of Islam is as varied as the regions in which Muslims live. The beauty of Islam is in its flexibility and allowance of cultural values to be incorporated into one's religious practice as long as they do not contradict Islamic tenets. Understanding Islam as practiced by a Muslim goes beyond acknowledging the sect or the type of *fiqh* (Islamic jurisprudence) that is followed. In addition to one's own unique life experiences, a Muslim's practice of Islam is also influenced by the intersections of (but not limited to) country of origin; culture; ethnicity; immigration; acculturation; Muslim identity; birth into or conversion to Islam; levels of faith, religiosity and spirituality; family relationships; multireligious families; and Islamic education.

Collaborative Language System (CLS)

CLS theorists contend that change is achieved through therapeutic, collaborative conversations, where the client defines both the problem and solution (Anderson, 2007). This postmodern approach to therapy not only values but incorporates the client's perspective of what is important and builds on her resiliency (Anderson, 2007). Previous researchers find CLS to be particularly conducive for integrating spirituality into family therapy (Blanton, 2002). Incorporating CLS within the CRT paradigm helps the MHP consider all appropriate contexts while allowing clients to remain the expert of their lives. Another primary goal of the CLS therapist is to provide a safe space for clients to explore and work through their therapeutic needs. Transparency of the therapist and sharing her own story, within appropriate bounds, is also encouraged as it enhances the therapeutic alliance and models vulnerability and openness for the client.

When a therapist shares her social location with the client, the client will have a better understanding of the perspective that is being offered in session. Having an open dialogue about the therapist's context will provide points of connection with the therapist, or create an opportunity to clear up any misconceptions. Additionally, having this conversation in the primary stages of therapy contributes to a client's decision regarding therapist fit. For example, because I am a *hijab*-wearing, second-generation, Bangladeshi-descended, Sunni, working, married woman with a child, a client can make many generalizations about my religious or therapeutic orientations. Having a dialogue regarding my worldview and my stance around differing perspectives may help demystify my position on sensitive social, religious, or political issues that the client may otherwise hesitate to bring up. Sharing perspectives or coming to a mutual understanding with the client can enhance the therapeutic alliance and client comfort. Conversely, therapist misunderstanding or insensitivity around such issues may contribute to premature termination of therapy.

Case Examples of Integrating Spirituality and Islamic Principles

As privacy and confidentiality are highly valued, and the Muslim community is well connected across the United States, in addition to changing clients' names, I pull from themes and discuss and combine examples from multiple cases to avoid providing specific details and risk possible recognition of clients.

Isthikhara

Ayesha came into session feeling hopeless about her relationship with her parents. She had come to a point where she moved out of her parents' house and into her own apartment. The decision to move out was very difficult due to parental expectations that the women in their family do not leave their parents' house unless they are married. She despaired about her conflictual and toxic relationship with her mother, worrying it would never get better. She felt that she was yet again failing her parents' expectations of her, which increased her sense of worthlessness.

In our sessions, she had been working on setting boundaries, and it took her a long time to make the decision to move out. I shifted her focus toward the strength needed to be able to choose a course of action that protected her mental health and well-being. She stated that *isthikhara* prayer, a special prayer that helps Muslims make decisions, played a huge role in her thought process. Ayesha described her deep connection to Allah and that throughout her life she always felt comforted when using the *isthikhara* prayer. I pointed out how special that connection was and that I was glad it was a source of support for her. She agreed that her relationship with Allah was unique because conversations she had with her peers revealed that similar feelings of connection and reliance on Allah did not come as easy to them.

When I asked her if she saw any blessings that resulted from the prayer, she began to describe having a sense of overall wellness, reduction in her stress and depression, and her mother actually being nicer to her on occasion. Since her connection to Allah was not only important to her but a source of strength and support, I told her I was reminded of the story of the Prophet (pbuh)—that his status as an orphan, having all caregivers pass away when he was younger, strengthened his bond with Allah. She stated that she did find a similarity in her life, that perhaps due to the lack of support from her parents, it was easy for her to find comfort and turn to Allah. After feeling revitalized by the sense of support and connection with her Creator, we concluded the session with a discussion about what it meant to have a relationship with her mother, and that although it may happen over time and in baby steps, it is possible with appropriate boundaries to establish a healthy connection with both parents. Subsequent sessions established strategies to reach that goal.

Evil Eye

Sarah came from a very traditional family that had strong beliefs regarding the concept of *nazr*, or the evil eye. They believed that anything negative that happens is the result of someone's envy and ill will toward them. Sarah reported that she unconsciously subscribed to that belief. She stated that she would catch herself automatically thinking about who gave her *nazr* when she would do poorly on an exam or had any relationship conflict. She wanted to be able to think about her problems differently so that she could begin to take more responsibility toward making improvements in her life rather than feeling helpless.

I initially responded to her concerns with empathy and validation as we discussed the history and role that this concept has played in her life. She also talked about the importance of Islam in her life and her connection to Allah. I asked her if she believed that the will and protection of Allah surpasses the human capacity to place *nazr* on others. When she reported believing so, I asked her if she could think of ways she could protect herself from *nazr*. She talked about reciting specific verses from the Quran, telling personal or important matters only to close people she trusted, and giving *sadaqa* or charity. Additionally, we discussed specific examples where she felt she may have been *nazr*ed, and I asked if she had to generate possible alternative explanations, what would they be. Through this process, which was initially difficult, she began to think about her issues differently.

Next, we delved into the alternative explanations and talked about the origins of her difficulties and relationship conflicts. As we slowly uncovered stories of traumatic incidents in her past and discussed relationships with her primary caregivers, it was easier for Sarah to see beyond *nazr*. She felt less helpless as we discussed possibilities for improving her relationships and steps she needed to take to reach her personal life goals. The more she worked toward her goals, the more she felt control over her life and less a victim of envious others. Since she mentioned that her relationship with Allah was important to her, our sessions also included discussions of her spiritual growth and journey. Our therapy sessions had inspired her to take a second look at other aspects of Islam.

She talked about how she was raised believing Islam had more to do with rules, and she has focused on protecting herself from Allah's punishment. She decided to take more classes, specifically regarding the attributes of Allah, and began embracing His other attributes of being merciful, loving, and a protector.

I asked if her new understanding of Islam influenced the way she viewed her life. After some thought, she was able to discuss all the different ways Allah had protected her with the combination of our earlier conversations regarding traumatic responses and how they can serve as protective mechanisms along with her new relationship with Allah, Sarah was able to see how Allah had protected her from remaining in abusive relationships. Whereas previously she was unable to assert herself and establish healthy boundaries, she was now able to spot red flags and avoid toxic relationships. Sarah also described several instances of Allah's mercy and blessings on her family. She discussed how although they were never very wealthy, they always had enough. She also talked about the valuable lessons her father taught her through his faith and patience. Her father never treated his extended family members poorly regardless of how they treated him. Sarah concluded that his good character and behavior brought more blessings upon their family.

DIVINE WILL

Mohammad's mother had passed away several years back from an unexpected terminal illness, and shortly thereafter his father was diagnosed with cancer. He had started to develop symptoms of OCD because his father was immunocompromised and he did not want to bring any illnesses into the house. Mohammad reported that he would wash his hands often and used hand sanitizer obsessively even on his phone. I had been working with Mohammad for several months at this point and helped him apply his spiritual strength and resilience to the issue of his OCD symptoms.

His initial complaint was about getting over his anxiety in talking to women to potentially marry. We discussed previous relationships of his that were emotionally abusive and led him to compromise his religious values. When I asked him about the role of religion in his life, he explained that it was always very important to him. His previous girlfriend was not Muslim but from *ahl-alkitab* (people of the book, i.e., Christians or Jews). He said that they got along pretty well for the most part, but she was embarrassed about him being Muslim, among other issues. She also did not appreciate his level of involvement with his parents. He believed it was his duty as a Muslim to care for his parents in every way possible and felt conflicted by her accusations of enmeshment. When his mother became ill he finally left the three-year relationship. We discussed how his relationship with Allah strengthened while his mother battled her terminal illness and how he accepted God's will when she passed away. He said he realized through this experience how much of his life is out of his hands.

We discussed how he worked hard to stay strong for the rest of his family, trying to be patient and accepting of God's will, but never felt he really had the opportunity to fully grieve his mother's loss. After thoroughly processing his grief, our conversations focused on highlighting his strengths, such as becoming the primary breadwinner and taking care of his entire family. We then searched for meaning behind his experiences, and he wondered if Allah was preparing him for handling greater difficulty in life. He knew that whatever it might be, he was definitely much stronger and more capable than he had ever been and fully embraced Allah's plan for him. I reminded him that with all he had gone through, his ability to rely upon Allah, his acceptance of *qadr* (God's will), and the realization of the limited control he has over his life and loved ones, would washing his hands excessively really prevent his father from getting sick? He responded by saying, "I keep thinking, *What if the one virus that I accidentally carry home is the one that ends up killing off my father?*"

In the spirit of transparency as encouraged by CLS theorists, I shared with him my personal tendencies to become obsessive about protecting my own daughter from getting ill and compulsively washing my hands. I told him a story about my travels to Mecca and Madinah when I took my five-year-old for her first *umrah* (religious pilgrimage) during the last ten days of Ramadan. A month before we left, my friend's two-year-old son had suddenly died of meningitis. In addition to witnessing this traumatic experience, my extended family told me to heed caution and asked, "What if your daughter gets sick or something happens because of the huge crowds?" The death of the little boy and all of the warnings I had received made my anxiety skyrocket, and hand sanitizer also became my best friend. On our trip, my heart palpitated when anyone sneezed or coughed, and I attempted to cover my child's face when we approached anyone who appeared sick. Nevertheless, as we shuffled through the crowds and prayed in the sacred mosque *Masjid Al-Haram*, I had an epiphany. I thought about how in this one place, there must have been people from every country on this planet who were also carrying viruses from all over the world. Here, millions of people were making *sujood* (prostration to the ground) in the same spot, coughing and sneezing in tight spaces for hours at a time. I concluded it could only be by the miracle of God that we were not dropping dead from disease. I could think of no statistical, scientific, or medical explanation of why we were not all sick, even though we were exposed to countless bugs from around the world. With that understanding, I felt relieved and that my daughter was being protected by Allah. I still had her drink *zam-zam* water (holy water), said prayers for her, and focused on worshiping Allah for the rest of the trip, but ultimately her protection came from God. By the end of our trip, my daughter did not have any symptoms beyond a common cold, and we returned home safely.

My story reminded Mohammad of a time when he was at the grocery store. He witnessed a woman sneeze into a box of fruit and place it back after she decided not to purchase it. At first he was outraged thinking what if he had purchased it, not knowing what had happened; he could have potentially killed his father. Then it dawned on him that there must have been hundreds of folks touching or sneezing on all kinds of produce and other items that he has bought in the past, but his father is doing just fine. He ended his story by saying he was okay with the things he could not control, but he just didn't want to be the person who brought home the virus that kills his father, especially if all it takes is for him to simply sanitize. I asked him that even if he did accidentally bring home a virus, wouldn't that be Allah's *qadr* for how his father dies? How much control do we really have when it comes to God's will? After a moment of silence, he agreed that the *qadr* of Allah is much more powerful than his actions and thanked me for the reminder. In subsequent sessions he informed me that he was able to reduce a large number, although not all, of his OCD symptoms as he left his father's fate in Allah's hands rather than his own.

GRATITUDE AND SPIRITUAL CRISIS

Having gratitude for the blessings bestowed upon a Muslim by Allah is an important concept in Islam. Many of my clients who have difficulty either conceiving children, getting married, finding or succeeding in a career path, or dealing with infidelity begin to despair and fall into a spiritual crisis. The despair is typically tinged with guilt and plummeting self-esteem. In this section, I highlight some of the questions clients ask themselves and how I address these questions in session. Some of these questions and thoughts include: "I don't understand why Allah continues to test me?"; "I know I have so much in my life to be grateful for, but I feel jealous when I hear about engagements or birth announcements. Then I feel guilty for being jealous." "I want what so many other people have. Why does Allah deprive me?" "Did I do something wrong that Allah is keeping this away from me?" "I must not deserve X, because I am not Y enough."

When clients suffer a spiritual crisis, I often begin by validating their perspective and give them ample time to process their feelings, especially those of loss and grief. If, and only if, the client is ready, I ask, "Is there anything at all that is going well in your life?" If clients themselves have made references to Islamic Scripture and find it helpful in our conversations, I may also incorporate the Quran or hadith (prophetic traditions) into the sessions. Typically the references will be paraphrased and couched within the context of my own experiences. This technique helps avoid pushing certain explanations or translations onto clients who may uphold differing Islamic perspectives. For example, in discussions around gratitude and blessings, I may introduce the idea of thinking about others who experience worse conditions or have greater struggles as the Prophet Mohammed (pbuh) recommends;

> On the authority of Abu Hurairah (رضي الله عنه) who said: the Messenger of Allah (pbuh) said: "Look at those who are beneath you and do not look at those who are above you, for it is more suitable that you should not consider as less the blessing of Allah."
>
> *(Bukharee 6490, abridged and in Muslim 2963 in its completion)*

Once I shared my story of a difficult experience I had raising my daughter. She was a high- needs, high-anxiety baby who slept very little and woke up every two hours for about two years. There were nights where I was utterly exhausted and depressed, and I could only think of how unfair it was that Allah had given other mothers happy babies who slept through the night as early as four months of age. On the nights when I felt I had nothing left to give to my child, I had to remind myself of a blog posting I read from a woman who lost her baby a few hours after delivery. She wrote a letter to tired, frustrated mothers saying that while she acknowledges how difficult it can be to lose sleep because of a crying, unrelenting child, she suggested that on the nights they needed motivation to keep going, they should think about the many women who lose sleep at night because they do not have a child or lost a child, and that they would give anything to stay up all night caring for one.

When clients interpret their struggles as a test from Allah, I take this interpretation as a signal to integrate an Islamic perspective into the therapy sessions. After referring to the hadith that states, "The Prophet (pbuh) said, 'When Allah loves a servant, He tests him' [*Tirmidhi*]," we search for evidence in the client's life of Allah's love as well as all the different ways Allah has protected the client from worse circumstances. Fathima, for example, had spent several sessions working on recovering from the trauma of past relationships. Moreover, she began to feel hopeless about finding a husband as her next birthday approached. She viewed her life as a series of tests from Allah and did not understand why she continued to be tested. After validating her sentiments and worries, I mentioned the above hadith, and we discussed all the ways Allah had loved her: blessing her with a successful career, a financially comfortable life, and a great relationship with her parents.

Integrating spirituality into therapy requires uncovering meaning behind struggle. Fathima's healing and spiritual growth came from discussions about how Allah protected her from horrible relationships in the past. She realized that although she was still single, she was certain that if she remained in her previous relationships she would have been miserable and divorced. After setting goals and appropriate boundaries, and discussing practical steps in helping her find a suitable partner for marriage, our sessions ended with a reminder of another important Prophetic tradition:

> The Prophet (pbuh) said, "No fatigue, nor disease, nor sorrow, nor sadness, nor hurt, nor distress befalls a Muslim, even if it were the prick he receives from a thorn, but that Allah expiates some of his sins for that." *(Bukhari 5641, 5642)*

Fathima shared that it gave her peace to think about Allah's mercy in this context and that her struggles were not in vain. Furthermore, she felt grateful for all the lessons she learned through her experiences and recognized how they have contributed to her strength and resilience.

SPOUSAL ROLES

During premarital therapy sessions, Omar and Khadija disagreed over what constitutes the role of primary breadwinner. They were preparing to get married and live in a multigenerational home with Omar's parents. Both partners used traditional Islamic tenets to guide their understanding of the spousal role and responsibilities. They believed a husband's role was primary breadwinner while the wife was responsible for household peace and child care. As a culturally responsive therapist with strong feminist views, I had to remain aware of my biases and be careful not to push my egalitarian values on the couple.

In these sessions, I worked within the couple's understanding of spousal roles and responsibilities. Khadija insisted that as primary breadwinner, Omar should cover the majority if not all of the household expenses. Omar argued it would make his parents feel uncomfortable if the couple abruptly changed the existing system of the household. He claimed his parents would feel more like guests or dependents of the couple if they would take away their major financial responsibilities.

I then asked Khadija why it was so important for her that Omar assumed these responsibilities. She stated that if her in-laws were carrying the burden of the financial responsibilities, she would feel that she is being taken care of by her in-laws rather than her husband, and that he would not be fulfilling his duty to her. Khadija mentioned in previous sessions that she planned on being a career woman and having children in the future as well. So the perspective I offered was one I had thought about myself as a working mother. I said to her, "You may disagree with me entirely, and that's perfectly fine, but I wonder if something that I had thought about in my own life would be useful for you two." I then talked about how if the responsibility of the wife is child care and she planned on having help from her in-laws and possibly day care when she had to work, it seemed that as long as the child is cared for, she is fulfilling her responsibility; moreover, it did not necessitate that she care for the child with her own hands. Likewise, if Omar was responsible for the financial needs of the family being met, would it be sufficient for him to make sure it was being taken care of, and not necessarily him needing to pay for all of the bills out of his own pocket? Khadija responded favorably to my thought process and stated that she had never thought about that perspective before and it made sense to her.

As far as their additional concerns about household structure, using the CLS paradigm, I focused on the language of the couple and how they were defining the role of primary breadwinner. I stated that it appeared that, for Khadija, the role of primary breadwinner also included being head of the household, and perhaps she envisioned their life with his family as the couple being primarily responsible for major household roles and responsibilities, while his parents, although still highly respected, would live comfortably with fewer responsibilities. For Omar, perhaps he envisioned more of the parents remaining in the same roles of household heads while the couple would adapt to living within the existing system. After presenting this summary, Omar was able to clarify his vision. He stated that he did see himself as head of the household but believed there should be a smoother transition in how the roles are shifted as the couple began taking the lead. He would feel more comfortable if his parents' financial responsibilities shifted slowly over a few years rather than taking it all away immediately after Khadija moves in. Khadija agreed that a slower transition would be an easier adjustment for everyone and she could agree to those terms.

Parenting and Kindness

A couple brought in their young adult son, Yousef, who was having trouble in school, establishing a career path, and holding down a job, and who suffered from low self-esteem. The parents complained that he was not very social and spent a majority of his free time in his room by himself playing video games. Typical of first-generation immigrant parents who come from collectivistic cultures, they came to the session with a barrage of complaints against their son. The more they spoke, the lower Yousef sank in his chair, looking at the floor and turning away from his parents. I then asked about his positive qualities, and while they had difficulty at first listing those qualities, they began to talk about his interest in politics, his respectful attitude toward adults, and how incredibly smart he was. Yousef's posture immediately changed; he faced his mother and appeared significantly more engaged. I asked his father if he noticed the difference in his son's posture. When he nodded his head, I explained that this is how we engage our children.

We discussed that while constructive criticism and rules are necessary, what is equally if not more important is the bond we create with our children. In their case, this bond would help establish his sense of worth and increase his self-esteem, which would in turn help him work toward a career path. Family therapy is strongly influenced by attachment theory, which I find to be congruent with Islamic tenets. Yousef's family identified as religious and active in the Muslim community, so when

Yousef's father told me that being affectionate with older children is not part of his culture, I felt safe enough to challenge this notion within an Islamic perspective. We spoke first about the loving nature of the Prophet Mohammed (pbuh) and discussed examples of his kindness and mercy toward children and people in general. I then brought up the manner in which the Quran was purposely revealed. The initial chapters functioned as a means to bring the hearts of the early believers closer to Allah and His Messenger. Once their faith and love were secured, the later chapters in the Quran focused more on establishing rules and regulations. In the same way, once we build a foundation of love and connection with our children, they will be more compliant with rules and expectations. A secure bond with primary caregivers can help them feel confident enough to venture out into the world, work within the rules of society, and eventually establish a successful career path.

COUPLES AND SEX

Contrary to popular misconceptions, within the boundaries of marriage, Islam is a sex-positive religion (Azam, 2013). A woman may even divorce her husband if she does not find him sexually attractive. Nevertheless, many Muslims come from cultures where sex and desire are considered taboo. Although Muslims are taught to have healthy sexual relationships with their spouses for both pleasure and procreation, typically nothing more is discussed regarding sex outside of rules pertaining to cleanliness. Based on the Muslim clients I have seen, the lack of open discussion and sex education contributes to their difficulty in this arena.

A couple who had been married for nearly a decade confessed that had they never had penetrative sex. Extremely shy in their demeanor, the couple explained that they were successful in pleasuring each other to orgasm but were unable to move beyond oral and manual stimulation. We talked in depth about their relationship quality and worked through the stress and depression the couple was experiencing, including despair about the possibility of never having children. I also thoroughly explored past sexual trauma with the couple until they felt the issue was resolved and ruled out its contribution to their sexual difficulties. The couple also mentioned that mental illness ran in the family, and they feared they may pass it on to future children. I wondered if their fears fueled their sexual dysfunction. I reminded them of their strengths as a couple and our discussions in earlier sessions about how as new immigrants to the United States they were able to overcome many obstacles and establish their successful careers. We spent several sessions thoroughly processing their fears and the couple was able to come to a point where they accepted God's will and were ready to deal with whatever may potentially be passed on to their child. With reliance on Allah for support, they decided that their desire to love and nurture a child outweighed their fears and worries.

Next, I recommended a visit to a gynecologist to rule out vaginismus and other physical dysfunctions. Eventually I invited the wife to explore herself and try to get comfortable inserting a tampon during the heaviest day of her next period (she had never used a tampon in the past). However, this exercise only increased her anxiety so I told her to stop immediately. In a session alone with her I asked her detailed questions about the times she and her husband attempted penis-vagina intercourse. She denied any sort of pain and explained she felt well lubricated and desired to have sex with him, but that "it just got stuck and wouldn't fit." After some serious consideration, I asked her to hold her hand in a fist and to squeeze her fist as tight as she could, then to try and put her finger into the tiny hole formed by her curled pinky. After doing so, I asked her if this was the same "stuck" feeling she felt during sex and she said, "Yes!" I informed her that her closed fist is similar to the condition of her vagina—that unlike the pictures seen in biology books, the vagina it is not a gaping hole where the penis slides right in. I then asked her to push her finger in as hard as she could until eventually her whole finger was inside her fist. I explained to her that this was similar to the first time a man and woman had penetrative sex. Especially at first, it would be slightly difficult to get through, a tight fit if you will, and may even be painful, but if she remained relaxed and allowed her husband to push himself, he would fit. She seemed to relax a bit but then became concerned about the pain. I replied that with sufficient stimulation and foreplay it should not be unbearable pain, especially since her gynecologist declared her to be physically healthy. I reminded her that she was a strong woman with a very high pain tolerance as she revealed in past sessions. In subsequent sessions, I decided not to bring up the matter unless the couple brought it up first, which they never did. Nevertheless, within a year or so after therapy termination, I received a birth announcement of their beautiful newborn.

Although Muslim clients can be shy and hesitant about discussing sexual matters, just like many non-Muslims can, it is important to provide a safe space in session to address such issues. More importantly, the therapist must be patient with clients until they are comfortable enough to open up about their sex lives. Not until our eighth session did the couple described here bring up the matter. I recommend being creative in your interventions and using the language of the client to increase comfort levels. As mentioned earlier, always remember that every Muslim client is unique, and comfort levels around the topic of sex can vary from extremely open to an absolute refusal to discuss it. For Muslims who appear uncomfortable, a matter-of-fact, medical/biological approach can be useful. Additionally, therapists can offer a reminder that during the Prophet Mohammed's (pbuh) time, women were so open regarding questions about their vagina that they would send him samples of their vaginal discharge. This reminder may help clients feel more open about discussing such topics (Syed, 2010).

Sexual Abuse

As a culturally responsive therapist, I mentioned above the importance of utilizing cultural consultants; those who have a deep understanding of a particular cultural, ethnic, racial, or religious group due to their membership within that group. Because openly discussing sexual matters may be taboo among many Muslims, I received an anonymous letter from a woman whom I will call Yasmeen, asking for help through a friend. Although this is not a typical therapy case, our correspondence beautifully illustrates the importance of input from a religious leader for this particular Muslim woman's journey to heal from past sexual molestation. I have seen clients who have had similar struggles, especially when attempting to reconcile their anger with the idea of forgiveness.

Yasmeen wrote that twenty years prior, when she was only a child, she had been molested for several years by an uncle. When she eventually told her mother after a few years had passed, her mother confronted the perpetrator and made him promise to stop, but she did so in private in order to protect his reputation. When the molestation continued, her mother finally threatened to tell the perpetrator's wife, at which point he did stop. Although Yasmeen was no longer being violated by her uncle, she was left to her own devices to process the trauma. Yasmeen had to pretend nothing had happened when she saw him at family gatherings, and her mother never said a word about it to her either. For many years, she relied on her faith and convinced herself that she was doing something noble by keeping the perpetrator's secret and protecting his marriage from potential dissolution. She thought she had moved completely past the whole situation until recently when another family member confessed she was being molested as well. Yasmeen wrote about unresolved feelings of anger and frustration, and despite working through them in therapy, her deepest concerns were about whether keeping the secret was actually the right thing to do according to Islam. Feeling torn, she worried that revealing the secret would "destroy" all the members of her uncle's nuclear family, but she also felt guilty and wondered if she was doing something wrong by keeping the secret. She did not understand why she was still so angry; she felt even guiltier when she realized she could not forgive him and secretly wished that Allah would punish him for what he did to her. She also mentioned if something like this happened to her own daughter, she would not stand for it and would protect her at all costs. She said she felt lost, and she hoped she could gain an Islamic understanding of the right thing to do and requested my advice. I clarified that I was not an Islamic scholar but that I would consult with one. As a CRT practitioner, I typically consult with a *sheikh* (scholar) or Imam of the client's preference, but Yasmeen stated that she did not have a preference.

My brother happened to be studying at Madinah University at the time and had access to a plethora of Islamic resources and scholars. I spoke with him about the matter, and as I waited, for his response I replied to Yasmeen with the following message:

> Unfortunately sexual abuse in the desi [Indian/Pakistani/ Bangladeshi] community occurs more often then we think. We live in a patriarchal culture that has been set up for centuries to protect men. Women are not only the victims but more often than not also the unconscious enforcers of this patriarchy. Ask yourself, what would the Prophet (phub) do if this was happening to his daughter? He would certainly not stand for it. You mentioned you would protect your daughter, no matter what. If as mothers we only have one part of the 99 parts of Allah's mercy, why would we think that Allah would be less merciful than us with His creation? And when people keep silent about such incidents they are giving perpetrators permission to continue molesting with little to no accountability.
>
> Our religion commands us to first and foremost stand up for what is right and forbid evil. Desi culture, on the other hand, values keeping peace, relationships, and reputation above all else. This collectivistic cultural value should not be confused with Islamic tenets. Furthermore, keeping silent is teaching future generations of women and girls that silence is the way to handle sexual transgression. Another question women should ask themselves is why do we value protecting the reputation/family of men who violate us over protecting our mental health, our marriages, and the future generation of women—not to mention other women who become prey?
>
> As far as I am concerned he destroyed himself when he made the decision to violate you, and his decision will bring upon him the consequences of his actions. Holding him accountable is a matter of protecting yourself, protecting other girls, and setting up the example for your daughter and other girls of how to deal with a situation like this.
>
> I'm pleased you are in therapy to help you process this mat-

ter. May Allah make it easy for you. Unfortunately, there are no quick or easy answers to a situation like this. It is something you have held on to for 20 years, and it will take time to process and overcome. Do remember that Allah's mercy has more depth than we can imagine and Prophet Mohammed (pbuh), the paragon of honesty and righteousness, exemplified the just treatment of women through his actions. If the perpetrator's family does fall apart, it is because of his decisions and his transgressions, not because you decided to stand up against his wrongdoings. Again I wish you all the best, and may Allah relieve you of your pain.

I told Yasmeen that I would have my response validated by an Islamic scholar via my brother and relay it back to her. After much research and discussions with experienced Imams, my brother reported that they agreed with my response. He mentioned that deep-rooted Desi culture interferes with a legitimate understanding of Islamic tenets. Desi culture, *not* Islam, dictated that she should stay quiet in order not to destroy the family, when in reality it was the uncle's transgressions that had the potential to do so. He stated that if it was still a problem, then the family should know about it and try to help the transgressing uncle stop molesting. In terms of forgiveness, Islamically speaking, the perpetrator needs to first sincerely feel sorry for what he did, repent, and ask for Yasmeen's forgiveness. At that point, Yasmeen has the right to decide whether she wishes to forgive him or not. Yasmeen has the right not to forgive him because he violated her, and she also has every right to expose him because it is probably better for the entire family to be aware of his actions, especially since the uncle is molesting others. My brother further explained that if they were living in a Muslim country, the perpetrating uncle would most likely be subject to capital punishment. My brother also mentioned that some Imams will typically suggest making a police report against the perpetrator. After relaying both my and my brother's responses to Yasmeen, she was extremely grateful and said they helped her better understand her own situation and assisted her in making decisions about how to move forward.

MULTICULTURAL/MULTIRACIAL COUPLE

Sumaiyyah, a born and raised Muslim of Arab descent, was planning on marrying Adam, a converted Muslim of African American descent. They struggled with gaining the acceptance of Sumaiyyah's parents. Sumaiyyah urged Adam to remain patient as her parents had a great deal of "cultural hang-ups" to work through regarding her marrying an African American man. He reported that he had been patient with her parents, had done everything they asked, called them on a regular basis, and had even provided documentation for proof of his income. Adam had difficulty understanding what "cultural hang-ups" they needed to work through. He also stated that he did not have high expectations; he was simply holding them to the standards of the Quran and *sunnah*. Sumaiyyah started to appear helpless as her validation efforts of his patience went in vain. I knew her sense of defeat came from the truth she was unable to verbalize. As the daughter of a first-generation immigrant myself, I understood her pain.

The Muslim community prides itself on Islam being forward thinking and having antiracist values. Muslim leaders and scholars often quote the following hadith: "Uqbah ibn Amir reported: The Messenger of Allah, peace and blessings be upon him, said, 'No one is better than anyone else except by religion or good deeds'" (Shu'b al-Iman 4767). Nevertheless, as much as it is denied, racism remains deeply embedded in the subconscious of the Muslim community. As a culturally responsive therapist (CRT) it was important for me to acknowledge this racism, and it was important for Adam to understand this as a systemic issue beyond Sumaiyyah's parents. I needed to say to Adam out loud the words Sumaiyyah could not articulate. I said to Yousuf that I could not imagine how he must have felt being rejected by Muslims, after being rejected by his own family for converting to Islam. I apologized to him on behalf of our community. I said that, as Muslims, we consistently fail to abide by our own Islamic values. We have failed to properly embrace converted Muslims, especially our African American brothers and sisters, and treat them with the acceptance and respect they deserve. Our *masjids* continue to be segregated by race and culture, and the younger generations that wish only to seek the blessings of marriage are faced with unnecessary obstacles. We have failed to take an active approach toward eradicating the racism that still exists.

However, I stated, I had hope that with increasing numbers of multicultural and multiracial marriages, and education- and social justice–minded second- and third-generation Muslims, the racism will decrease. In the meantime, they should remain empathic toward and be a source of support for each other. I applauded the couple for taking the more difficult route of seeking acceptance from Sumaiyyah's parents through patience and appropriate boundaries, rather than deciding to cut them off entirely. The couple was further relieved when I related stories of other multiracial couples I knew personally who felt real acceptance from their families over time, especially as grandbabies came into the picture.

Challenges

Embracing the philosophical paradigm of the CLS model helps me avoid contention with clients. CLS and CRT position clients to be the central driving force behind therapy sessions as the therapist works within their worldview. Any perspective I may offer to clients, as illustrated above, (1) comes from a place of sharing, (2) comprises suggestions that have been helpful for me and others, and (3) can be accepted or completely rejected by clients as they deem appropriate. CRT requires MHPs to be mindful of their biases and take great care to avoid impressing their values on an unsuspecting client.

Challenges have been few, but they exist nonetheless. One such challenge I have come across in my work is when clients begin to rely heavily on me for answers or to "fix" their issues. Psychotherapy is a Western practice that has evolved from Western countries. Muslims who are not from Western countries are accustomed to visiting religious or community leaders to acquire *nasiha* (advice). They may also view MHPs similar to primary-care physicians or other medical doctors and expect them to be experts who can provide them with answers they need. In these scenarios I typically address the issue by explaining early on in the process and limits of therapy, and how I can be helpful.

Another challenge I have come across is when a client wants to use me as an authority figure to back or further an agenda. For example, a client may say, "You are a Muslim therapist, so tell my *X* that Islam says Muslims have to do *Y*," where *X* is a wife, husband, child, teenager, and so on, and *Y* is whatever agenda the client wishes for me to further. With one couple I counseled, the husband brought a page of quotations from Islamic Scripture and was ready to back up his arguments if needed. He leaned far more to the traditional/conservative side of Islam compared to his wife and believed that my role as a Muslim therapist was to bring more Islamic tenets to the table that would reinforce what he thought was the correct way to resolve their disputes. To address this situation, I asked the husband if using Scripture and Islam to persuade his wife to act in certain ways has worked in the past. If it had not worked for him thus far, then it probably would not be the most effective course of action in therapy either. He agreed that expecting different results from the same actions did not make sense. I offered instead to help the couple listen to each other's perspective and Islamic understanding and try to create a compromise that was amenable to both parties. Setting the stage for therapy allowed the couple to be receptive to working in subsequent sessions on issues pertaining to respect, expectations, and cultural differences.

Recommendations and Ways Forward

MHPs who wish to integrate spirituality into their sessions with their Muslim clients should be aware of the varying levels of spirituality and religiosity among potential clients. MHPs should allow clients to guide the correct course of action and level of spiritual integration. I suggest using the following indicators to bring religion or spirituality, or both, into the discussion:

  ▸ If clients quote or refer to Islamic Scripture

- If clients refer to their situation as the result of or related to Allah's test, mercy, or punishment
- If clients are on a quest to find meaning behind their struggle
- If clients ask existential questions and are searching for greater purpose in life, and
- If clients specifically sought out a Muslim therapist to ask for an Islamic perspective

I have had many other Muslim clients for whom religion or spirituality were the least of their concerns—not because they were not spiritual or religious but simply because they did not find it relevant to their issue at hand. Their purpose for seeking out a Muslim therapist was to have their cultural context understood. As mental health professionals we should continue to create space for conversations around spirituality that are meaningful and relevant to the client. This approach will help provide CRT to a marginalized population that may be cautious about this unfamiliar yet valuable resource.

References

Anderson, H. (2007). The heart and spirit of collaborative therapy: The philosophical stance—"A" in relationship and conversation. In. H. Anderson & D. Gehart (Eds.), *Collaborative therapy: Relationships and conversations that make a difference* (pp. 43–59). New York: Routledge. https://postmoderntherapies.wikispaces.com/Collaborative+languaging+therapy

Azam, H. (2013). Sex, marriage, and eroticism in contemporary Islamic advice literature. *Journal of Middle East Women's Studies, 9*(1), 54–80. doi:10.2979/jmiddeastwomstud.9.1.54

Blanton, P. G. (2002). The use of Christian meditation with religious couples: A collaborative language systems perspective. *Journal of Family Psychotherapy, 13*(3–4), 291–307. doi:10.1300/J085v13n03_04

Seponski, D. M., Bermudez, J. M., & Lewis, D. C. (2013). Creating culturally responsive family therapy models and research: Introducing the use of responsive evaluation as a method. *Journal of Marital and Family Therapy, 39*(1), 28–42. doi:10.1111/j.1752-0606.2011.00282.x

Syed, S. (2010). Quandry of female vaginal discharge: Pure or impure. https://muslimmatters.org/2010/09/22/quandary-of-female-vaginal-discharge/

Integrating Islamic Spirituality into Psychodynamic Therapy with Muslim Patients

Ibrahim Rüschoff, MD, and Paul M. Kaplick, BSc

The authors wish to thank Sadiya Khalid for professional English editing and Malika Laabdallaoui for helpful comments on an earlier version of the manuscript.

Overview

ISLAM HAS BEEN a part of diverse cultures throughout its history and is deeply entrenched in the traditions of these cultures. In the long term, this will also apply to the West, where Islam has started to establish itself: first, through large-scale migrations after the end of the colonial era, and second, through later labor migrations. Islam has evolved as the second largest religion in the world after Christianity and will continue to be well immersed in the cultural heritage of the societies of its followers, particularly in the West.

Muslim psychologists and psychotherapists globally are an integral part of the psychosocial support structures of their societies. They not only pursue a theoretical interest in how they can embed their own religious tradition in the legacy of psychology but they also emerge as key figures capable of answering questions based on psychotherapy for Muslim patients, who understand their religion as an all-encompassing way of living and who demand to see their religion considered in therapy (Kaplick & Rüschoff, 2018).

This chapter initially sketches out the legal and practical framework of psychotherapy in Germany and then briefly outlines opinions on psychoanalysis and psychodynamic therapy in the Islamic psychological literature. We proceed by examining how Islamic spirituality can be integrated into the practice of psychodynamic therapy, which we exemplify in four case studies. Taken together, such integrative work meets Islamic and professional requirements, we argue, and can be consolidated in a meaningful therapeutic concept.

Psychotherapy in the German Health System

Psychotherapeutic support for German society is housed in the country's medical care system. A maximum number of possible physicians and psychotherapists in a certain region is determined by the Ärztliche Selbstverwaltung/Physicians' Self-Regulation, which also processes payments for health insurance companies. The overwhelming majority of patients are medically insured, and only couple and family therapy needs to be paid for privately. Treatments exceeding fifty hours require a report to be sent to a reviewer, who assesses the symptomatology, etiology, and intended therapy. Health insurance in Germany covers cognitive behavior therapy, analytical psychology (C. G. Jung), and psychoanalysis (Sigmund Freud, Alfred Adler) and its derived psychodynamic therapeutic practices.

CASE STUDIES

Case studies presented in this chapter were gathered from a private practice in a small city near Frankfurt, Germany, with about sixty-three thousand inhabitants and a relatively large number of Muslims. The foundation of therapeutic work in this private practice is psychodynamic therapy, a derivative of psychoanalysis. The practice accommodates two therapists, one male medical and one female psychological psychotherapist, both of whom provide therapy for approximately sixty to seventy patients. Patients are seen on a weekly basis for two years on average. Treatment takes place in a face-to-face setting while seated.

Most patients speak German, but one of the therapists is also fluent in Arabic and Tamazight (a Berber language spoken in northern Morocco). Roughly 80 percent of the patients have a Muslim background, and most of them can be considered as practicing, observant individuals; 70 percent are women, mostly ages twenty-five to sixty. Most diagnoses are depression, anxiety, and trauma, predominantly associated with family and marital conflicts, as well as work-related problems. Symptoms are often displayed in relation to religion, in particular to parental and marital conflicts, but also, for instance, expressed as the anxiety of not having lived Islamically enough and to suddenly stand in front of Allah in the event of death.

Psychoanalysis and Psychodynamic Therapy in the Islamic Psychological Literature

Traditionally, there has been a certain degree of hostility in the Islamic psychological literature toward theories and concepts revolving around psychoanalysis and psychodynamic therapy (Amer & Jalal, 2012; see Abdul Razak & Hisham, 2013; Badri, 1979, 2012; Shah, 2005). However, such work appears to predominantly build on the theories of founding father Sigmund Freud and arguably disregards most of the diverse theoretical traditions of his successors. Fortunately, publications (e.g., Abu-Raiya, 2014; Skinner, 2010) and conferences, such as the Islamic Psychoanalysis / Psychoanalytical Islam conference convened by the College of Psychoanalysts in June 2017 in Manchester, United Kingdom, have facilitated a constructive cross talk between Islam and psychoanalysis in recent times. Some of these activities have contributed to an illumination of the great potential of psychoanalysis for the psychotherapeutic support of Muslim patients. Here, we extend this line of research with the argument that psychodynamic therapy specifically provides an appropriate basis for the incorporation of Islamic spirituality in the healing process of Muslim patients.

Ibrahim Rüschoff, MD, and Paul M. Kaplick, BSc

Exploring the Integration of Islamic Spirituality into Psychodynamic Therapy with Muslim Patients

Requirements of an Integration of Spirituality into Psychodynamic Therapeutic Practices

According to the German guidelines of psychotherapy, psychodynamic therapy encompasses, "etiologically oriented therapeutic approaches, which treat unconscious psychodynamics of currently operating neurotic conflicts and structural disorders, while considering transference, counter-transference, and resistance. A concentration of the therapeutic process is pursued through limitation of the therapeutic goal, primary conflict-centered intervention, and restriction of regressive processes" (Federal Joint Committee, 2017, p. 12).

In this chapter, we rely on the framework of psychodynamic therapy and focus on psychoanalytical object relations theory in its most recent forms (Donald Winnicott, Ana-Maria Rizzuto), rather than on Freud's original views. This framework proposes that the child's access to the world and its people is shaped by the child's relationships to early persons of reference, as the child fulfills basic needs for attention, contact, and to be held (Heine, 2007). As such, the ability to form relationships constitutes the fundamental element of the conception of human nature as propagated by object relations theory.

A novel understanding of the central notion of *illusion* has recently contributed to a mainly positive attitude toward religion. While Freud depicted religion as an illusion that humankind had to surmount during its process of maturation, today's object relations theory conceptualizes illusion as a key human characteristic that "accompanies [humans] throughout their life and enables them to give life meaning and form, beyond its mere existence" (Santer, 2003, p. 198). This meaning and form include creativity, play, culture, and also religion.

From an Islamic perspective, humans are born with *fitra*, an innate, primordial orientation toward Allah (Mohamed, 1995; Skinner, 2010), and are always and above all *relating to someone*. Moreover, humans, as opposed to instinctual animals, have to learn relationships. This learning takes place during early childhood, predominantly in the family, and underlines the importance of early objects and persons of reference (Doering et al., 2017). Therefore, early experiences of relationships critically determine social relations and patterns of relationships in the long term, which take effect not only with respect to parents, family, and the environment but also toward Allah. This situation is influenced by patriarchal family and societal structures and, Islamically, by the tight intertwining of the parental relationship and Islamic texts. The texts include specific Quranic verses (e.g., 17:23; 46:15) and the Sunna (prophetic tradition), such as the prophetic saying that paradise lies under the feet of our mothers.

Frequently we experience a situation of diverging opinions between parents and their children, causing disrespect and, therefore, sinful behavior. This situation regularly possesses serious consequences for a person's self-image as a Muslim and the person's religious practice. As a further exemplification, a depressive patient who suffered from severe feelings of guilt and maintained a problematic relationship with his irascible and unpredictable father got to the heart of the problem by concluding, "If my father gets exasperated with me, then *I* have committed a sin." He realized the implausibility of his statement only later in therapy.

Defining what *Islamic* actually entails is crucial for comprehending the possibility of building an Islamically integrated psychodynamic therapy on the grounds of object relations theory. We propose to adhere to a wider understanding of Islam, such as that proffered by Tariq Ramadan (2001). Ramadan advocates that there is *only one* Islam, yet its realization requires the consideration of societal circumstances that mold the way Islam is lived. As such, accomplishments of various societies do indeed belong to the human heritage and cannot be disregarded by Muslims: "In the area of social affairs (*Muaa'malaat*), all means or instruments, traditions, arts and clothing, which do not in themselves or through their usage contradict Islamic tenets are not only acceptable but *per definitionem* Islamic" (Ramadan, 2001, pp. 245–246).

Furthermore, we postulate that the truth is only with Allah as the Quran testifies on many occasions (e.g., 5:48; 22:69; 32:25). Therefore, any opinion expressed by humans, including those of the most distinguished scholars, is eventually *one* perspective and relative; there has been a broad consensus on this view in Islamic history (Bauer, 2011). On applying this notion to psychotherapy, we arrive at the conclusion that one particular therapeutic school of thought cannot be *always* right or *always* wrong. Instead, each school embodies a specific treatment approach and constitutes a variably appropriate and abstract "map" for the real "landscape," the patient, to achieve a distinct therapeutic goal (Buchinger, 1995).

This view gains even more in importance when appreciating the prevailing agreement in academic literature that a therapeutic relationship is crucial for accomplishing therapeutic goals (Lang, 2003; Staats, 2017). The Islamic concept of man and understanding of human nature adopted by the clinician, and the resulting attitude toward the patient, are of paramount significance in therapy. Such conception of Man acknowledges the patient's innate relationship to god (*fitra*) and the self-responsibility of humans for their actions. Adopting these views results in attitudes of empathy, respect, understanding, and acceptance of the patient by the therapist.

Numerous scholars early on in Islamic history pondered the nature of human beings and their psychic life. A prominent example is Abu Hamid Al-Ghazali (1058–1111 AD). He conceived a model of human nature that still stimulates and guides psychological works of contemporary researchers and practitioners. This model describes the relationship between the *ruh*, *'aql*, *nafs*, and *qalb*, whose interaction is essentially distorted in several disorders and can be employed to evaluate therapeutic outcome on a long-term basis (Abu-Raiya, 2012).

We have so far delineated a top-down theoretical approach that aims to integrate Islamic principles into one stream of "Western" psychotherapy. This appears to be meaningful and promising from various angles:

- ▸ Muslim psychotherapists are bound to professional standards and are part of the medical and psychotherapeutic support system of a society. This precludes any inclusion of parapsychological elements into the therapeutic practice such as exorcism and prescribing amulets. Patients, including those who are Muslim, expect results- and goal-directed practice grounded in the most recent research.

- ▶ The extent of integrating Islamic principles into therapy requires an alignment with the religious attitude of the patient and, therefore, needs to be flexible.

- ▶ We argue that psychotherapy is, due to a variety of social factors, culturally shaped and that there is no *one and only* Islamic therapeutic approach. A psychodynamic therapeutic form of treatment, which empowers patients to perceive their own conflicts through introspection and also to address and sort out relationship conflicts in regard to important persons of reference, may prosper in Europe and the United States. Yet, in other cultures, such an approach may malfunction or be entirely useless, and other treatment forms and therapeutic strategies may be imperative (Kakar, 2012).

- ▶ Psychotherapeutic approaches stemming from Western culture are not per se un-Islamic, materialistic, and impractical, as we have illustrated above in the broader definition of what *Islamic* entails. Such an understanding reaches beyond theoretical accounts that are directly derived from the Quran and the Sunna.

- ▶ The top-down approach works. Symptoms of patients have eased, and the results of a top-down-oriented practice are appealing, even from an Islamic viewpoint: Therapy does enhance their ability to engage in relationships to their parents, themselves, and Allah. It enables many patients to attain a fulfilled Muslim life. They develop a comfortable, personal, and responsible relationship to God; sense His mercy; and live their Islamic life wholly and not merely because of their fear of punishment from God.

What Is "Islamic Spirituality"?

There is no universally accepted definition of spirituality. A core, bare-bones definition of it that we prefer to use was distilled by Bucher (2014), who pledges for a "broad understanding of spirituality whose center is attachment, on the one hand, horizontally with the social environment, nature, and the cosmos and, on the other hand, vertically with the all-encompassing ultimate, holy one, for many still god, who is beyond human grasp" (p. 69). Because of the manifold forms of expression of spirituality across different cultures and religions, it has to be appreciated that Islamic spirituality manifests in the middle of life and is not part of a reclusive attitude: "The body was solely created for the purpose of serving the soul in exercising its function and fulfilling its duties and responsibilities. The body is not imprisoning the soul but is its workstation and fabric; if the soul grows and develops, then it is through this workstation. Therefore, this world is no place of punishment, detaining the unfortunate soul, but a field to which God has sent it in order to work and to fulfill its duties toward him" (Maududi, 2017). If the world is the workstation of the soul, the therapist of a Muslim patient is practically always confronted with the question of spirituality. "He who has a 'why' to live for can bear almost any 'how'" (Nietzsche, 2017, p. 7). This statement from the German philosopher Friedrich Nietzsche elucidates the role of the question of meaning in life. As we know that nothing occurs without Allah's will, the question of meaning is an access point to spirituality, especially for Muslim patients. If God tests us with sorrow, conflicts, and problems, what does he want from us? What does he want to reveal to us? What is the ground he wants to lead us to?

THERAPEUTIC GOALS

Based on the aforementioned frame of reference, we briefly tackle here therapeutic goals that should be discussed and defined together with the patient. It is useful to act with sound judgment as the complexity of some encountered problems and limited therapy contingents necessitate for a restriction of therapy to those who experience the most restraints in their everyday life. Three essential therapeutic goals emerge for Muslim therapists.

First, the patients want their symptoms (e.g., depression or anxiety) to go away, which is why they sought therapy, and this is realizable in the context of psychodynamic treatment. In contrast, more deep-seated personality developments and changes require a long-term, high-frequency therapy such as psychoanalysis.

Second, as illness always restricts a person's freedom (e.g., sudden uncontrollable anxiety attacks, severe drive disorder) and disables the ill person despite major efforts to pursue vital actions, extending the degrees of freedom for the patient should be the therapist's chief concern. Given that the patient gains in freedom and can increasingly exercise autonomy in one's experience and responsibility, the treatment likewise permits living up to the patient's responsibility toward God and facilitates a godly life, which therapists should wish for the patient but cannot impose on him/her.

Third, and a goal broader in scope, is that the therapist should aid the patient in coming close to a state of *Al-Nafs Al-Mutmainna* (the tranquil soul; 89:1), while being well aware that this state is like a star that provides orientation but can ultimately not be reached, except by the prophets. The status of a tranquil soul is that which went to great lengths and knows of its own strengths and weaknesses, which holds responsible only itself for its own shortcomings (i.e., waives any projection and endures reality), and which rests in its center and whose will is in accordance with Allah, and such a status is supposed to be the highest stage of human development. Controlling for the therapeutic outcomes takes place in a nonstandardized manner through

- Evaluation of the reduction of symptoms;
- Resolving dysfunctional behavioral and relationship patterns;
- Enhancing the subjective well-being of the patient
- Evaluating the ameliorated degrees of freedom in regard to the world and the patients themselves and, thus, advancing the self-responsibility for their own Islamic life.

THE ROLE OF THE THERAPIST

In light of the importance of the therapeutic relationship for therapeutic success, particular attention should be directed at the therapist's role. Specifically, fostering one's own spirituality as a therapist has an immediate impact on therapy, making it an integral part of the therapeutic relationship. In all modesty, the therapist ought to appreciate that he/she is a mere instrument of Allah ("And when I am ill, it is He who cures me";

, 26:80), through whom Allah provides the patient his *rizq* (supply). To cope with the religious and psychological insecurity and the un-Islamic behavior of the patient, the therapist is in need of his own stable stance and settled convictions. That is the only way to maintain inner peace as a therapist and to deal, in attending distance, with the transference of the patient and the therapist's own countertransference.

Challenges of Integrating Islamic Spirituality into Therapy

Most Muslim patients come to our private practice because it was brought to their attention that it hosts Muslim clinicians who take their religious practice seriously. The patients hope to be understood and to not be put in a place to explain too much about their own religion and culture. Some have had unfortunate experiences with certain therapists' Islamophobic attitudes and critique that some therapists have solely emphasized Islam and the Islamic lifestyle of their patients as the source of all difficulty or completely disregarded their religion, even though it makes up a significant portion of the patient's life.

Having said that, some patients seek therapy because their problems are related to religious matters as the question of meaning is strongly connected to their daily life as a Muslim and Islam as their lifestyle. For instance, patients report that, in absence of any apparent reason, they experience extreme feelings of guilt toward their parents or children. Others state being depressed because they cannot pray or that they are subjected to the behavior of an aggressive spouse who maintains inappropriate relationships with the opposite sex, not knowing how to respond in an Islamically correct manner. Further examples include patients who cannot sense the mercy of Allah and, as a result, encounter feelings of loneliness and anger. Many link symptoms with the possession of *jinn* (supernatural creatures) or *sihr* (magic) and have already consulted an Imam whose recommendations to increase supplications and recitation of Quran and to be patient seem to have failed.

Upon gaining diverging experiences with non-Muslim therapists, patients commonly expect something uniquely "Islamic" in therapy, something they can recall from their local mosque or from conversations with an Imam. Furthermore, patients seek explanations of their problems and concrete advice, and how exactly to deal with these problems from their general practitioner. Taking into account that non-Muslim therapists presumably leave most of the spiritual aspects of the patients' problems unattended, Muslim therapists can blunder into a different trap: tending to easily identify themselves—overtly or unconsciously—with their Muslim patient, idealize them when they behave Islamically, or devalue them when they openly sin. Therefore, for therapy to prosper, sustaining a professional attitude that, under no circumstance, abandons a supporting therapeutic relationship will be critical.

Muslim patients show a tendency to rationalize their anxiety of change with "Islamic" arguments and look for endorsement from their Muslim therapist. However, theological discourse does not belong in therapy. The question "I am allowed to demand submissiveness from my wife, right?" is of a legal (fiqh) nature and to be dealt with by an Imam. As therapists, we have to address such questions solely in a psychological manner, seeking prior problems with the spouse in question that may have triggered the question in the first place. Similarly, for a patient who experiences separation anxiety and who handles the symptoms with Islamically justified control, the response must be interpreted to enable the patient to face the anxiety. Answering the question "What is it really about?" only allows *one* reality, namely the *psychological* one; however, it is important to acknowledge that, in the patient's defense, for the patient there is also a religious meaning and hence several realities in "What else is it about?" Psychological problems can only be solved *psychologically* and not *legally*.

The same logic applies to the question of truth, which is a *theological* question and, in the same way, cannot be solved psychologically. Whether someone is possessed by a *jinn* or held under a spell does not, ultimately, play a significant role in therapy. In the situation at hand, when the patient addresses this topic, it is a *psychological* reality and both therapist and patient may collectively examine ways to clarify the underlying problem from a psychotherapeutic viewpoint.

Local traditions are frequently justified as Islamic and, in effect, are practically untouchable, such as the social interaction with parents or children. In such cases, we avoid a discussion of right or wrong but present alternative narratives from the Quran and Sunna.

Case Study 1: "Will I Still be Your Daughter even When I Disappoint You?"

A young woman raised in a family of Arab civil war refugees who came to Germany in the 1990s presented with depressive and anxiety symptoms. She observed the headscarf at the beginning of her therapy and greeted with the traditional Islamic salutation, "*As-salamu alaikum*." Aside from her symptoms, she reported openly on her drug use and frequently changing sexual partners, with whom she was involved in sadomasochistic practices and erotic massages—which she traded for money ever since puberty—while simultaneously yearning for an Islamic family.

During the anamnesis, it became apparent that the young woman had been raised with a rigorous parenting style, strictly propagating the adherence to Islamic tenets. Her parents admonished her incessantly to behave righteously and suggested that she would not be part of the family anymore if she disobeyed the parents' moral orders. This built up a strong defense, making it impossible for the patient to engage peacefully in *dua* (supplication) or to recite Quranic verses, which she had prevalently pursued when her mother was around.

The patient could have easily chosen to go to any psychotherapist, yet she explicitly sought out a Muslim practitioner. Also, she correctly inferred the negative attitude of her *Muslim* therapist toward her sexual behavior, though not overtly communicated, at the very start of the therapy. This was an important early signal that the choice of a *Muslim* therapist, to whom she could confess her Islamically inappropriate sexual behavior, served an important function, and its utilization was crucial for therapeutic success.

At some point during the therapy, she aired her astonishment that the therapist did not discharge her from psychotherapy because of her "misbehavior," and that he continued to bear with her. The therapist liked the patient and obviously was aware of her sins. However, there was, likewise, a strong awareness of her adversity, her desperate search for *unconditional* acceptance, her rebelling against her parents ("So I will behave the way you always exemplified bad behavior!"), and her anxiety that her family could find out. The fact that a male Muslim therapist, the "father," unconditionally accepted her regardless of her Islamically inappropriate behavior was key to the treatment. It proved to her that the therapeutic relationship did not have a price and that she could be the way she wanted. Therefore, reporting on her sexual behavior lost its function.

After several years of therapy, her depressive and anxiety symptomatology eased. She earned a degree, is now working full-time, has not had contacts involving sadomasochistic practices for a long time, and can only picture sexuality in a stable relationship. On reflection, Islamic matters were barely discussed during therapy; the emphasis was more on her work-related and social situation, which, by now, has stabilized. In recent times, the relationship to her parents has gained importance, and it can be assumed that an enhancement of the patient's autonomy, in particular with regard to her mother, has facilitated the search for her own Islamic lifestyle.

This case signifies the role of Muslim practitioners in psychodynamic therapy. The psychodynamic of the patient would have—presumably—not functioned properly in the absence of a Muslim clinician. He essentially enabled the patient to make corrective emotional experiences. Furthermore, this case illustrates that evaluating the patient's behavior as inappropriate and actively attempting to redirect it would have mirrored the behavior she encountered from her parents. Such a response would have confirmed her idea that being accepted only comes with the price of adaptation to the expectations of others, and she would have probably terminated therapy prematurely. On applying the observed case to family life, we conclude that adolescents can behave in an Islamically inappropriate way, but they nevertheless do remain the parents' children—even though such behavior is difficult to tolerate and may evoke many conflicts.

Ibrahim Rüschoff, MD, and Paul M. Kaplick, BSc

Case Study 2: An Imam's Panic Disorder

A thirty-five-year-old Imam of a small mosque sought therapy because of increasingly severe panic attacks. Such attacks had initially been present during his previous *hajj* (pilgrimage) when he circumambulated the *Kaaba* (the cube at the center of the mosque in Mecca). When leading prayers at his local mosque, he could only recite short *surahs* (chapters of the Quran) and had to quickly complete the prayer to gain control over the emerging panic attack, which had already attracted attention among community members. Worse yet, it was only with the greatest difficulty that he was able to perform the Friday prayer, which lasts for about forty-five minutes, including the sermon. As a leader of his community, he was repeatedly exposed to the critical glare of the public and almost grew unable to practice his profession. However, these problems did not appear at home.

The patient descended from a small Egyptian village and was the prize pupil of the local Imam of that time—to an extent that he selected him as his potential successor. In the context of this small Egyptian village, such selection was a great honor and built the pride of his stern yet beloved father who reiterated the commitment of his son.

Although the patient did indeed aim to become an Imam, he aspired to study at a well-known madrassa and did not want to spend his life in the intellectual milieu of his village close to the margin of subsistence. At the age of seventeen and against the will of his father, he (and a friend) applied to a prestigious madrassa that was one thousand miles away and was accepted. Just before the signing of the madrassa contract, he had a severe panic attack that forced him to return to his village. He pursued his studies in an alternative, smaller madrassa closer to his home, which allowed him to enjoy his vacation in his village. Upon graduation—before his father passed away—he got married and relocated to Germany, where he obtained a job as an Imam in a mosque. His community appreciated his kind nature and admired his modern opinions.

The described panic disorder exemplifies a psychodynamic that can be observed equally in non-Muslim patients but is, in this case, entirely housed in a virtually closed Islamic environment. This was because of his role as an Imam who had barely interacted with people of other faiths or no tradition at all, for instance, at the workplace. The panic disorder progressed along with an autonomy conflict in the relationship with his father, which was characterized by a strong, religiously justified obedience that was amplified within the milieu of the small Egyptian village. Though the act of disobeying his father by means of signing the contract for his study program at the faraway madrassa did not materialize because of his first panic attack, the problem had not been eradicated as he continued to reject the wishes of his father and of his Imam to pursue his studies within the village.

During his pilgrimage, when he visited the *Kaaba*—the house of God "the Father"—being practically inside the lion's den, his psychological defense collapsed under the pressure of his unconscious fear of punishment, and the symptomatology persisted. Therapeutically, it was critical that the Muslim therapist accepted the patient's disobedience in the evolving father transference and liberated him through widening his understanding of diverse religious viewpoints on parental obedience from his experience of sinful action. Furthermore, the therapist enabled the patient to affirm his marriage and relocation to Germany as well as his occupation as an Imam as a chance for his personal development and his whole family that would have never been possible in his village. A trusting therapeutic relationship between the patient and the therapist quickly developed, the symptomatology ceased, and when the patient successfully completed his therapy, he pursued his work as an Imam without any constraints. He spent his next vacation in Egypt, where, after years, he was even capable of praying in the mosque of the small village in which he was born and raised and where his father had socialized" (Rüschoff, 2017, pp. 107–108).

Implementing the Integration of Islamic Spirituality into Therapy

The religious practice of Muslims is as diverse as that of Christians or Jews. It plays a significant role in the life of Muslims, and that is why it has to be appropriately considered in therapy. Religious topics should be prioritized to an extent that corresponds with the religious profile of the patient. To assess the importance of religion in the patient's life, a spiritual/religious anamnesis history can help to address the religious attitude and the intensity of religious practices, for example, whether the patient prays, reads the Quran, fasts, and the general character of religious everyday life. This also includes an appraisal of the patient's beliefs about the etiology of his or her symptoms. In our subjective experience, roughly 20 percent of our patients independently attribute their symptoms to *jinn* and *sihr*, and 40 percent suspect such an influence upon query. Such anamnesis should take place without any judgment from the therapist.

An inclusion of Quranic verses, hadith (prophetic sayings), and examples from the Sunna may take place after the religious anamnesis and after clarifying that the patient benefits from such interventions, and moreover, that including religious elements will not provoke resistance or lead to a withdrawal from therapy. Particularly relevant Quranic verses for therapy are as follows:

- "Then do ye remember Me; I will remember you." (2:152)
- "O ye who believe! Seek help with patient perseverance and prayer: for God is with those who patiently persevere." (2:153)
- "On no soul doth God place a burden greater than it can bear." (2:286)
- "He said: 'With My punishment I visit whom I will; but My mercy extendeth to all things.'" (7:156)
- "He hath inscribed for Himself [the rule of] Mercy." (6:12)

Quranic verses that convey an extended context of meaning in therapy seem to be associated with parental images when evaluating patients' statements. However, examples from the *sira* (prophetic history) that establish a practical and eternal realization of rather abstract Quranic principles in daily life serve as role models. This specifically applies to topics pertaining to ideals of masculinity, handling marriage, and raising children. The prophetic role model steadily gives Muslim patients the courage to overcome anxiety and to probe insights gained through therapy in daily life. This is equally relevant for women, who can benefit from great examples such as the lives of Khadijah or A'isha, as well as ordinary women who approached the Prophet regarding intimate and familial problems. Referring to these role models ensures that newly developed relationship patterns will be seen from an Islamic context— which is commonly denied in traditional views on masculinity in social structures such as mosques or families (Rüschoff, 2017).

ALLAH'S NINETY-NINE NAMES AS KEY TO THE PSYCHODYNAMICS OF A DISORDER

Practicing Muslim patients experience symptoms (e.g., depression, anxiety, and compulsions) every now and again as an expression and outcome of a lack of *iman* (faith) and of their own religious practice that is believed to be insufficient. They do pray, regularly read the Quran, fast, honor their parents, and are known in their community for their piety and for their just behavior. Nevertheless, they are permanently afraid of the anger and the punishment of Allah and worry they have not done enough to attain paradise. Others despair because they do not feel the mercy of God or are suicidal. Still others resign from religion altogether, thinking that they cannot please Allah, and then lapse into depression, have a constant fear of failure or feelings of worthlessness, or grapple with uncontrollable/impotent rage, which is frequently directed toward the immediate social environment and causes suffering in families. In this context, many patients do not directly see the point when the therapist expresses an interest in their childhood rather than their actual acute problems.

Object relations theory has provided evidence that early experiences of relationships have a strong impact on believers' later image of God (Rizzuto, 1979; Heine, 2007). Parents are the initial representatives of God and His omnipotence, which is why many patients exhibit typical behavioral patterns and emotional reactions toward Allah as shaped by their experiences of relationships in early childhood and closely resemble them. This yields a therapeutic approach that not only has a positive effect on the patients' relationships in the here and now but also on the internal images of their parents and, therefore, also on the one of God and the Islamic lifestyle enjoined by him. In therapy, this

Islamic lifestyle is, therefore, achieved *per effectum* and not *per intentionem* (Frankl, 2004). The latter falls within the area of activity of an Imam who can provide a form of Islamic chaplaincy that gives clear directions on Islamic behavior.

To elucidate this association between problems with religion and God and their relationship with his or her own life experiences, psychodynamic therapeutic sessions, which comprise a maximum of one hundred hours in Germany, can utilize Allah's ninety-nine most beautiful names (*Asma' Allah Al-Husna*) to illustrate God's characteristics in a reasonable period of time. Patients are presented with a German and Arabic list of these names and are asked to mark twenty characteristics that touch them and bear emotional meaning to them, even if it's unusual. A couple of names such as *Al-Rahman* (The Most Merciful) or "*Al-Ghafur*" (The Much-Forgiving), are checked most of the time, presumably because of their prominence. As for the remaining names, most of the patients cannot rely on learned content but have to make personal choices. Names such as *Al-Hasib* (The Bringer of Judgment), *Al-Darr* (The Harmer), *Al-Mumit* (The Bringer of Death), or *Al-Muntaqim* (The Avenger) appear on such lists. While discussing these lists in the following therapy session, many patients are surprised by their selection and ascertain that their choice mirrors those characteristics that they attribute to their parents and that they love, oppose, fear, or wish for themselves. Insights into these connections represent, for most of those who associated their symptoms with a low level of *iman*, on the one hand an immense relief. On the other hand, it increases their motivation for change with the help of insights that this therapy is helpful beyond the consultation of an Imam, who can indeed enhance their despair by simply asking them to make a greater effort.

CASE STUDY 3: THE FEAR OF FAILURE AND
ALLAH'S NINETY-NINE NAMES

A thirty-five-year-old man of Kurdish origin who was born and raised in a secular family in Germany complained of strong mood swings. He easily plunged into hopelessness and depression, while reporting the urge to be steadily active and to complete every task immediately and to perfection. If he did not do so, then he felt severe restlessness and would start to perspire.

Difficulties associated with religious practices provoked the patient to seek therapy. He was proud to be Muslim and started practicing the religion about one year before the onset of psychotherapy. He was well versed in Islamic texts and displayed painstaking accuracy in his adherence to religious precepts. At the same time, he noted severe anxiety toward making mistakes. If he missed *fajr* (early morning prayer), the entire day seems to be ruined to the core for him, and recovery before the evening became unfeasible. He only had a few social contacts and was reluctant to frequently visit the mosque as he did not get along with any of the other visitors, and people were talking about him. He reported the steady urge to correct the wrong behavior and the attitude of everyone in the mosque, including the behavior of the local Imam, if he was under the impression that someone performed something religiously erroneous—no matter how negligible it may be—as he did not want to be a "partner in crime."

The patient was puzzled that the therapist assessed his biography and could hardly imagine that his problems were deeply rooted in his past. Descriptions of his childhood depicted his mother as a very active person whose demands he could never meet. She was unsatisfied with him and always compared him to others, in particular his uncle, toward whom the patient developed a serious disliking. His father was to him "like a stranger" from whom the patient never felt loved and who envied and rejected his son, who was a creative thinker and built tricky and complicated constructions as a young child and was admired for his inventiveness. The patient's father labeled him as mad when he constructed a reverse gear on his scooter as a sixteen-year-old, which the patient described as the end of his relationship with his father.

The treatment used the described list of Allah's ninety-nine names. Strikingly, he did not select a single, warm characteristic of Allah— not even *Al-Rahman* (Arabic: the Most Gracious), which almost every patient picks. Instead, the patient picked names like *Al-Muntaqim* (The Avenger) *Al-Darr* (The Harmer), *Al-Hakam* (The Judge), *Al-Raqib*(The Watchful), and *Al-Muhaymin* (The Controller). Attributes like *Al-Alim*(The Knowing) or *Al-Muqqadim* (He Who Brings Forward) had a negative connotation to him, as these were associated with achievement and instigated his fear of failure. A detailed discussion of the list with the patient yielded his own surprise at his selection. Comparing those of Allah's characteristics that he attributed to his parents with those that he wished from them nourished his insight and understanding that his fear of failure, and in particular the associated problems with religious practices, were not rooted in his religion but in his relationship with his parents and the internalized images that he projected on God.

Dealing with Jinn and *Sihr*/Magic

As already briefly addressed above, roughly 20 percent of our patients suggest a possible connection between their problems and the influence of *jinn* and 40 percent agree on such a connection upon direct request. This helps patients explain their problems in a cultural and religious frame of reference that provides guidance and, therefore, security. Most of them have seen an Imam who did confirm a possession, but whose treatment did not lead to a significant improvement. Muslims do accept the existence of *jinn*, and Muslim therapists should address these issues with patients, but they should likewise discuss and explore alternative causes that can elicit a self-activity for healing in a therapeutic context. Therefore, it is therapeutically crucial to accept those explanations but to leave them with the patient and to provide other psychological perspectives on the problem (Khalifa & Hardie, 2005). If the patients sense that the therapist accepts their perspective of things as one of several possible explanations, then the therapist's alternative explanation is also plausible for the patient and the therapy, which leads to an improvement of the symptomatology and a good therapeutic outcome despite diverging opinions (Rüschoff & Laabdallaoui, 2011).

CASE STUDY 4: MARITAL PROBLEMS AND JINN POSSESSION

A thirty-five-year-old man presented with anxiety symptoms and stated insecurity in the presence of close relatives, which had persisted since he got married four years before his therapy commenced. Anxiety about losing his wife seemed to reoccur, and he therefore tried to control her. During the two previous years, he suffered from two panic attacks and attributed these, as well as his anxiety-related and marriage problems, to the influence of *jinn* and magic. The patient descended from the southeast of Turkey where he lived with his mother until he turned thirteen. He fostered an intensive relationship with her. His father was working in Germany, pursued an authoritarian and bossy parenting style, and did not tolerate any disagreement with him, even to this day.

Due to an error of the physician who conducted his circumcision in Turkey, it happened that his penis was very short. Out of concern that, because of his short penis, he could not have a happy marriage with any woman, he married his cousin with whom he nurtured a close friendship during his childhood and who, he figured, would not leave him upon discovering his shortcoming. The wedding night was a "catastrophe," and sexuality practically did not materialize during the first few months of marriage. During the ensuing months, he turned increasingly aggressive, hated his wife "like the devil," and was unable to stay at the marital home. Because of his abnormalities, and only on the insistence of his wife, they sought help from a local Imam. The Imam diagnosed the influence of several *jinn* and magic that aimed at separating the couple and applied various rituals upon which their problems noticeably ceased—and which constituted the proof for everyone that the problems were due to *jinn* and magic.

From the perspective of psychodynamic therapy, the sense of insufficient masculinity and the severe anxiety about ultimately being deserted by his partner were defended in the guise of an unconscious testing of their relationship by means of extreme aggression toward his wife. Relying on traditional interpretative patterns, this phenomenon was explained through the influence of *jinn* and harmful magic. Corresponding rituals, the patient's stance of his wife, a rehabituation of the couple toward each other, and the resulting decreasing anxiety of loss led to an easing of the situation.

This therapy centered on liberating the patient from the exceedingly tight relationship to his mother and to simultaneously behave as a Muslim man without falling back into the role patterns he learned from his father. With the help of a caring and securing therapeutic relationship, unconditional appreciation, and examples from the Quran, *sunna*, and *sira* (life of the prophet), the patient developed a growing security in interacting with his work colleagues, became an active member of his local mosque, and set limits on the behavior of his parents. Previously they put him under financial and moral pressure with continuous reference to his Islamic duty to obey his parents. Concurrently, he accepted a job offer that allowed him to move into a more spacious apartment. Finally, he even underwent urological treatment that, after two operations, enabled normal sexual intercourse for the first time. His life has proceeded harmoniously, and the couple now has two children.

During the last phase of his successful treatment, the patient's beliefs in the etiology of his problems and symptoms were addressed. He ascertained that the "psychological map" not only made more sense but he also realized that, after all, it first allowed for accessing a successful change. Before that, he felt like a helpless victim of *jinn* and magic and less than a man capable of acting. The security imposed by the Muslim therapist who ensured that the patient's actions were Islamically legitimate provided additional strength.

Conclusion and Outlook

The experience with daily therapeutic work reveals that the integration of Islamic spirituality into therapy provides proper functionality. We argue that a deep theoretical penetration into the wide field of Islam and psychology is of utmost importance (Kaplick & Skinner, 2017). Further development in this area can enhance standardization of therapeutic techniques. While we propose that there is not a *one-and-only* Islamic approach with clearly delineated treatment methods resulting from a defined set of theoretical presuppositions (an Islamic take on human nature, etc.), there ought to be an integration of available theoretical and practical concepts that are compatible with Islamic precepts and that may also involve slight adjustment—as is the case for object relations theory. Following Heine (2007), object relations theory can only outline the formal frame of reference, whereas religions are required to provide contextual input. As such, Rizzuto restricted the validity of her inquiries on the development of God representation to the religiosity of the Christian world: "I will not attempt, in this study, to extrapolate conclusions to other cultures, where other beliefs and religious systems provide a different God or representation of God. The Eastern world in particular, requires another study suiting its cultural traditions" (Rizzuto, 1979, p. 221). Spero (1992) has contributed to the integration of object relations theory and Judaism, and Finn elucidated its applicability to Buddhist thought (Murken, 1998). Based on this body of literature, we must prospectively sketch out the possibilities and limitations that object relations theory poses for understanding Islamic spirituality and therapy for Muslim patients.

References

Abu-Raiya, H. (2012). Towards a systematic Qur'anic theory of personality, *Mental Health, Religion & Culture*, 15(3), 217–233. doi:10.1080/13674676.2011.640622

Abu-Raiya, H. (2014). Western psychology and Muslim psychology in dialogue: Comparisons between a Qur'anic theory of personality and Freud's and Jung's ideas. *Journal of Religion & Health*, 53(2), 326–338. doi:10.1007/s10943-012-9630-9

Amer, M. M., & Jalal, B. (2012). Individual psychotherapy/counseling: Psychodynamic, cognitive-behavioral, and humanistic-experiential models. In S. Ahmed & M. M. Amer (Eds.), *Counseling Muslims: Handbook of mental health issues and interventions* (pp. 87–118). New York: Routledge.

Badri, M. (1979). *The dilemma of Muslim psychologists.* London: MWH London.

Badri, M. (2012). Why Western psychotherapy cannot be of real help to Muslim patients. *Sudanese Journal of Psychiatry*, 2(2), 3–6.

Bauer, T. (2011). *Die Kultur der Ambiguität: Eine andere Geschichte des Islams* [The culture of ambiguity: A different history of Islam]. Berlin: Verlag der Weltreligionen.

Bucher, A. (2014). *Psychologie der Spiritualität* [Psychology of spirituality]. Weinheim, Germany: Beltz.

Buchinger, K. (1995). Wissenschaftstheoretische Grundlagen der Psychotherapie [Philosophical scientific foundation of psychotherapy]. In O. Frischenschlager, M. Hexel, W. Kantner-Rumplmair, M. Ringler, W. Söllner, & U. V. Wisiak (Eds.), *Lehrbuch der Psychosozialen Medizin. Grundlagen der Medizinischen Psychologie, Psychosomatik, Psychotherapie und Medizinischen Soziologie* [Handbook of psychosocial medicine: Foundations of medical psychology, psychosomatics, psychotherapy, and medical sociology] (pp. 775–790). Vienna: Springer.

Doering, S., Hartmann, H. P., & Kernberg, O. (2017). *Narzissmus: Grundlagen— Störungsbilder—Therapie* [Narcissism: Foundations—disorders—therapy]. Stuttgart, Germany: Schattauer.

The Federal Joint Committee / Gemeinsamer Bundesausschuss. (2017, Sept. 16). *Richtlinie des Gemeinsamen Bundesauschusses über die Durchführung der Psychotherapie* [Legal guidelines of the Federal Joint Committee on the implementation of psychotherapy]. https://www.g-ba.de/informationen/richtlinien/20/

Frankl, V. (2004). *On the theory and therapy of mental disorders: An introduction to logotherapy and existential analysis*. London: Routledge.

Heine, S. (2007). In Beziehung zur Welt im Ganzen. Der Ertrag der Objektbeziehungstheorie für Theologie und Seelsorge [In relation to the world as a whole: The earnings of object relations theory for theology and pastoral care]. In I. Noth, & C. Morgenthaler (Eds.), *Seelsorge und Psychoanalyse* [Pastoral care and psychoanalysis] (pp. 108–121). Stuttgart, Germany: Kohlhammer.

Kakar, S. (2012). *Kultur und Psyche. Psychoanalyse im Dialog mit nicht-westlichen Gesellschaften* [Culture and psyche: Psychoanalysis in dialogue with non-Western societies]. Gießen, Germany: Psychosozial-Verlag.

Kaplick, P. M., & Rüschoff, I. (2018). *Islam und Psychologie in Großbritannien, den USA und Deutschland: Gegenwart und Zukunft von institutionellen Strukturen muslimischer Psychologen* [Islam and psychology in Great Britain, the United States, and Germany: Current and future institutional structures for Muslim psychologists]. *Wege zum Menschen, 70*(1), 79–89

Kaplick, P. M., & Skinner, R. (2017). The evolving Islam and psychology movement. *European Psychologist, 22*(4), 198–204. doi:10.1027/1016-9040/a000297.

Khalifa, N., & Hardie, T. (2005). Possession and jinn. *Journal of the Royal Society of Medicine, 98*, 351–353. doi:10.1258/jrsm.98.8.351

Lang, H. (Ed.). (2003). *Wirkfaktoren der Psychotherapie* [Power factors of psychotherapy]. Würzburg, Germany: Könighausen & Neumann

Maududi, A. A. (2017, September 24). *Das islamische Konzept der Spiritualität* [The Islamic concept of spirituality]. http://www.islamreligion.com/articles/10033/islamic-concept-of-spirituality/

Mohamed, Y. (1995). *Fitrah and its bearing on the principles of psychology. American Journal of Islamic Social Sciences, 12*(1), 1–18.

Murken, S. (1998). *Gottesbeziehung und psychische Gesundheit. Die Entwicklung eines Modells und seine empirische Überprüfung* [Relationship to God and psychological health: Development of a model and its empirical examination]. Münster, Germany: Waxmann.

Nietzsche, F. (2017). *Götzen Dämmerung—oder wie man mit dem Hammer philosophiert* [Twilight of the idols]. Hamburg, Germany: Nicol Verlag.

Ramadan, T. (2001). *Muslimsein in Europa. Untersuchung der islamischen Quellen im europäischen Kontext* [To be a European Muslim]. Köln, Germany: MSV Verlag.

Rizzuto, A. M. (1979). *The birth of the living God. A psychoanalytic study.* Chicago: University of Chicago Press.

Rüschoff, I. (2017). *Religiöse Ressourcen in der Psychotherapie muslimischer Patienten* [Religious resources in the psychotherapy of Muslim patients]. *Spiritual Care, 6*(1), 103–110. doi:10.1515/spircare-2016-0206

Rüschoff, I., & Laabdallaoui, M. (2011). *Djinne, Zauber und "Böser Blick"—Psychodynamik und Umgang mit traditionellen Krankheitsvorstellungen bei muslimischen Patienten* [Jinn, magic, and "evil eye"—Psychodynamics and interaction with traditional ideas of disorders amongst Muslim patients]. In T. Heise (Eds.), *Integration, Identität, Gesundheit. Beiträge zum 5. Kongress des DTPPP in Klagenfurt 2011. Das transkulturelle Psychoforum* [Integration, identity, and health. Proceedings of the Fifth Congress of the DTPPP in Klagenfurt: The transcultural psychoforum]. Verlag für Wissenschaft und Bildung, Berlin: 131–139.

Santer, H. (2003). *Persönlichkeit und Gottesbild. Religionspsychologische Impulse für eine praktische Theologie* [Personality and the image of God: Religious psychological impulses for a practical theology]. Göttingen, Germany: Vandenhoeck & Ruprecht.

Shah, A. A. (2005). Psychotherapy in vacuum or reality: Secular or Islamic psychotherapy with Muslim clients. *Pakistan Journal of Social and Clinical Psychology, 3*(1–2), 3–20.

Skinner, R. (2010). An Islamic approach to psychology and mental health. *Mental Health, Religion & Culture, 13*(6), 547–551. doi:10.1080/13674676.2010.488441

Spero, M. H. (1992). *Religious objects as psychological structures. A critical integration of object relations theory, psychotherapy and Judaism.* Chicago: University of Chicago Press.

Staats, H. (2017). *Die therapeutische Beziehung. Spielarten und verwandte Konzepte* [The therapeutic relationship: Varieties and allied concepts]. Göttingen, Germany: Vandenhoeck & Ruprecht.

CHAPTER 6

Family Therapy and the Use of Quranic Stories

Rabia Malik, PhD

IN THIS CHAPTER I describe how I have tried to integrate Quranic stories with systemic psychotherapy theory (more commonly known as family therapy) as an intervention in my work with Muslim clients. I outline aspects of my journey, what drew me to systemic therapy, and my interest in working with Muslim clients, as well as how I have modified systemic theoretical ideas and practice to include Islam. I illustrate this with a case example, where I used the Quranic story of Abraham and Ismail to explore a mother and son's relationship. Finally I consider the question of integration—the possible bridges and areas of tension between Western psychotherapies and Islam.

My Background

My interest in Islam and psychology developed out of my doctoral research on the cultural construction of depression among Pakistanis (Malik, 2000). My focus had been on the intersection between culture and psychology and how mental distress may be expressed and experienced differently across cultures (Kleinman & Good, 1985). While studying this topic, I realized that underlying the cultural beliefs of my first-generation migrant Pakistani informants was an Islamic metaphysics more akin to the assumptions in *tibb* (Islamic medicine; Khan, 1986). Characterized by a more holistic orientation in which mind, body, and spirit are connected, individuals are not regarded as bounded entities separate from their environment, but rather more permeable and interconnected in relationships, and where the notion of self and agency is closely connected to a relationship with God. This was born out in my informants presenting depression with more somatic and not just psychological symptoms, with them seeing the causes as having to do with their relationship with God and a moral universe and family relationships, rather than primarily with them individually. The first port of call for treatment subsequently was also seeking spiritual healing, followed by turning to family and then medical professionals. The importance of these underlying cultural and religious contexts in understanding people's explanatory models of mental health and illness drew me to systemic therapy.

Although systemic therapy emphasizes the importance of context, like other therapies it still has not always deeply engaged with the cultural and religious context and different meaning systems (Krause, 2007). In recognition of this, the Marlborough Family Service—a mainstream child and adolescent mental health service in the U.K. National Health Service (NHS) in the 1990s set up a specialist service for ethnic minority clients, with the remit of developing culturally appropriate therapy to engage local communities that were not accessing mainstream mental health services at that time (Krause & Miller, 1995). I had the privilege of working within this service and later leading it for a number of years (Malik et al., 2009). Although the main focus was on cultural difference and providing therapy in the clients' mother tongue, after September 11, 2001, we started receiving clients who were asking more specifically to see a "Muslim therapist," and so the markers of identity seemed to be shifting.

My own interest in religion and spirituality had been growing since my doctorate, and I had begun studying with some Muslim scholars, asking questions that were pertinent to my work and finding ways of applying what I learned in my work with clients for whom religion was important. This raised for me a whole set of questions about what it meant to be labeled as a "Muslim therapist" and what clients meant and expected when they asked to see one. So started a journey into explicitly integrating Islam into my work. Like with all therapeutic work, I needed to start with my own self-exploration and my relationship to Islam and the Muslim community. I had been brought up a Muslim but had questioned many aspects of religion and especially what I saw as the inconsistencies I observed in the Muslim community around me. After my father died, I had been reminded of my faith and wanted to reconnect with God and religion from my own deep yearning and desire for something more truthful.

The first client I saw who had specifically asked to see a Muslim therapist was instructive in helping me understand the role religion may play in psychotherapy. Initially, I had felt somewhat self-conscious in responding to this request, as the client was an Egyptian man who was suffering from long-term depression. I am a Muslim woman who does not wear a *hijab*, and distracted by these social markers of whether I looked "Muslim enough." I wondered if this might be a barrier for him in engaging with me. To my surprise, in the first session, the client mentioned nothing about Islam. He talked about his long-standing depression that had been triggered by losing a number of his family members in Egypt when a building they lived in collapsed. He had seen the whole tragedy unfold, and since then he had been depressed and unable to continue with his day-to-day life. Unclear about why he had specifically requested a Muslim therapist, I asked him why this had been so important to him. He responded by saying, "I want to talk about my depression, not Islam," which confused me further. So, I continued my work with him over a few sessions, keeping his original request in the back of my mind, and then one day as we talked about what he had witnessed he broke down and said, "I feel angry with God. Why did He let this happen?" I understood then why he had requested to see a Muslim therapist, as at some subconscious level, when he referred himself, he knew that his relationship with God and his religion were significant in what he wanted to talk about.

I engaged with his questions, and we explored why "bad things happen" and our feelings of helplessness and anger and how faith is tested in the face of such tragedy and loss. The important learning point for me in this work was that, at times, mental health was foregrounded, with his religious beliefs in the background, and vice versa, and that they were interconnected in the way that he made meaning of his difficulties. For many Muslim clients, being able to explore their relationship with God and religion is vital in overcoming their difficulties since it is commonly an integral part of their worldview, even if be it subconscious, and what is meaningful to them.

Since then, I have been trying to find ways of integrating religion into my clinical practice; building bridges, modifying models that I use from within the systemic psychotherapy field, as well as developing new techniques and ways of asking questions that fit with the Islamic paradigm. I have been fortunate enough to meet Islamic scholars who have had a deep understanding of the human condition and inspired me and guided me in this work. The trainings I received with them have made me challenge many of my own taken-for-granted beliefs and patterns, as well as helped me find new meanings and ultimately deepen my own faith, which in turn has been invaluable in developing my psychotherapy practice. I describe later how I have done this with the use of Quranic stories in particular to explore family relationships.

Systemic Psychotherapy: An Overview

Systemic psychotherapy emerged in the 1950s in reaction to dissatisfaction with psychiatry and psychoanalytic thinking, with their almost exclusive focus on the individual and a heavy emphasis on pathology. Systemic psychotherapy took a more interpersonal approach and examined the role of communication in the development and maintenance of severe disorders, such as schizophrenia, and suggested the usefulness of bringing family members together to talk and collectively intervene with difficulties (Burnham, 1986). Early pioneers influenced by developments in the fields of biology and mathematics on feedback patterns and self-regulation applied general systems theory and cybernetics to human interaction and relationships (Bateson et al., 1956). Rather than seeing events in a linear sequence, cybernetics proposed that causation was a continuous dynamic circular process, taking place over time, thus making it harder to pinpoint blame and attribute cause or individually pathologize. Hence, understanding the contexts of interpersonal relationships and emerging patterns became important in understanding and intervening in the problem. This included the cultural context. The early anthropological work of one of the founding fathers of systemic therapy, Gregory Bateson, was very much influenced by this broad approach to understanding human interaction (Krause, 2007). However, like most psychotherapies, systemic therapy has developed largely along Western ethnocentric lines. The dominant and normative models of relationship patterns remain based on Western kinship structures and Cartesian mind/body dualism that has characterized Western medicine and therapy since the European Enlightenment. These differ significantly from Islamic metaphysics and the more holistic cultural approach that is found in the Muslim world. I return later to Bateson's work and vision, as I think they contain the possibility of taking a much broader and more radical approach to systemic psychotherapy, bridging culture, and interest in the "sacred," which he wrote about in the later part of his life (Bateson & Bateson, 1988).

Systemic therapy did make more advances in addressing issues of power and diversity in the 1970s and 1980s under the influence of postmodernism and the turn to what is referred to as "second-order cybernetics." Postmodernism challenged the modernist endeavor, namely that reality is potentially knowable and the idea that there is a "truth" that we can discover. It questioned the assumption of "objectivity" and laid bare the "subjectivity" of the therapist. It shifted the focus from the observation of patterns and processes alone to socially constructed beliefs and personal meanings, especially as mediated through language, including those of the therapist. Hence the cultural context and the therapist's own culturally biased views came to the foreground, primarily through feminist critiques. Dallos and Draper (2000) argue that the psychotherapist as observer draws distinctions, and this is not just an epistemological act but also a political act, hence encouraging therapists to become more self-reflective and also potentially opening systemic therapy up to different social constructions or worldviews. This shift enables one to understand and argue that unless the therapist has explored his or her own cultural and religious beliefs, the therapist may be limited in the ability to engage with Muslim clients (or clients from other cultures or faiths, for that matter) and to intervene in ways that are meaningful to their socioculturally constructed beliefs and views of reality (Yon et al., 2017).

Coordinated Management of Meaning

As outlined above, the shift to second-order cybernetics and language in systemic therapy led to a growing focus on the construction of beliefs, patterns, and ultimately meaning. The Coordinated Management of Meaning (CMM) model developed by Cronen and Pearce (1985) is a good model for illustrating the complex interaction of different contexts and the role of communication in the coordination and management of meaning between people. I outline this theory briefly and in a somewhat simplified manner, with the main purpose of showing how the religious context in relation with the cultural, familial, and individual contexts may play a role in any given episode in the management of meaning, and then, through a case example, how Quranic stories can be used as interventions.

CMM theory (Cronen & Pearce, 1985) was used by systemic therapists to help understand what was going on in practice in any moment of interaction and to guide intervention. According to CMM, we construct our own social realities through communication and social interaction. This is not just a passive process of perceiving messages but rather is a socially interactive process that involves creating coherence and coordinating the way we manage meanings with other people and in the context of relationships at the macro (sociocultural) as well as micro (familial and individual) levels. The theory proposes that we establish certain rules that guide our actions. These are constitutive rules, such as how behavior should be interpreted or what meaning it has in a given context, as well as regulative rules such as what behavior a person should undertake next. The three key tenets to CMM are coordination, coherence, and mystery.

Cronen and Pearce (1985) suggest that meaning is organized in a hypothetical hierarchical manner with embedded contexts that confer coherence across levels, so that meaning at any level can be understood in the context of a higher level.

Coherence refers to the management and organization of meaning—the process by which we tell ourselves and others stories to interpret

Coordinated Management of Meaning

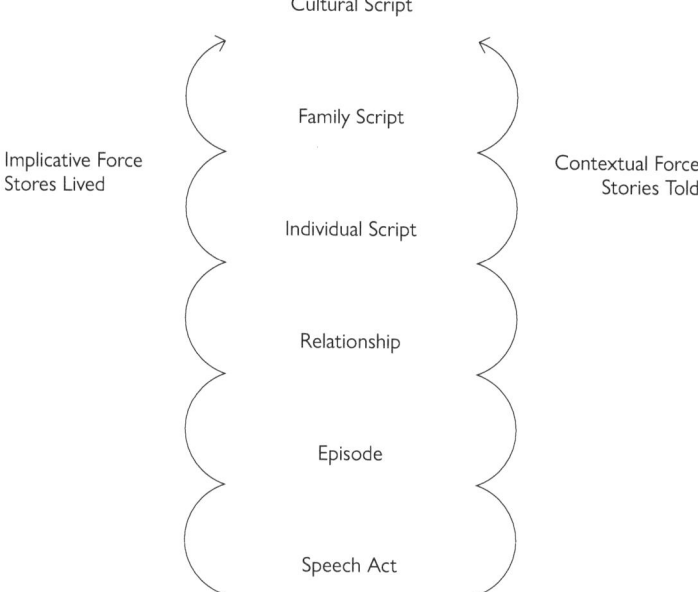

Cultural Script

Family Script

Implicative Force
Stores Lived

Individual Script

Contextual Force
Stories Told

Relationship

Episode

Speech Act

the world around us and our place in it. These can be referred to as *scripts.* To elaborate on this, from a bottom-up approach, any behavior or speech action can be understood in the context of the episode in which it occurs; the episode can be understood in the context of the relationships between those involved; the relationships can be understood in the context of the individuals' life script, which can be understood in the context of the family script; and the family script can be understood in the context of the prevailing cultural script/beliefs and so on, so that each level is influenced by the level above. When these "stories told" are interpreted in the same way by others, we have coherence—for example, if what is considered good or bad is agreed upon collectively.

Cronen and Pearce (1985) regard the higher levels as exerting a stronger contextual force downward, sometimes referred to as dominant "stories told," or we can think of this in other words as forming the social expectations on us. We tend to coordinate—that is, attempt to fit our actions with those of other people to reproduce coherence and dominant patterns. In other words, we try and make our stories lived fit with the stories told and lived by others. This does not necessarily mean we have mutual understanding with or like or agree with the patterns we produce (Pearce, 1999), but we have a tendency to want to share meanings as it helps us develop a sense of common understanding. However, the commitment to coordination may not go smoothly, and coherence isn't guaranteed. Pearce (1999) argues that we often in fact live in the tension between the stories we tell others and ourselves and the stories we live with others. "This tension is the source of much of the joy and pain of human life" (Pearce, 1999, p. 12) and often the reason people seek therapy. If we want to create change, it may be necessary for us to contest and challenge stories told. Working from the bottom up, we can exert a weaker implicative force upward on the basis of stories lived or our experiences. This implicative force tends to be weaker than the contextual force, as it often means going against dominant familial and cultural stories. However, it can become stronger, through communication and perhaps psychotherapeutic intervention, and thereby the meaning of levels can change and coherence and coordination can be renegotiated.

Cronen and Pearce (1985) stress that the relationship between levels is not fixed, but rather is circular, dynamic, and reflexive, and meaning is always emerging. But at any one time all of these contexts are interacting and impinging on one another in the meanings we construct sometimes unexpectedly. This they refer to as "mystery"; beyond stories told or lived there are always other possibilities. Pearce (1999) argues that language is a two-edged sword. In creating one picture of reality, for instance, it predisposes us to see reality in that way rather than in all the other ways in which we might have seen it; in interpreting our motives for acting in one way, we obscure all the other ways in which we might have understood a particular event. In fact, interestingly, he refers to the Tao Te Ching to make his point:

> The way that can be described is not the eternal Way.
> The name that can be named is not the eternal Name.
> That which cannot be named is the eternal reality.
> Naming is the source of all particular things.

The number and nature of levels is also not fixed, but in systemic therapy we tend to use the six levels, as in the diagram to understand what is going on in family interaction. In my work with Muslim families, I have found it helpful to introduce a seventh level, which is the religious or ethical context. I think this is important, as for many of the migrant families I work with, as previously argued, religion is an important marker of difference and part of their everyday understanding of life.

Religion or ethics also presents a higher context that has the capacity to help us contextualize and challenge culture. I believe that for second-generation children of migrants, religion has become a way of challenging both: cultural and familial practices that do not always fit within the current cultural context in which they now live, as well as the wider mainstream socially limiting scripts of race and culture, thereby enabling them to negotiate their identity and break out of hegemonic discourses. Of course, the religious context can be liberating but also limiting. I have found that if the religious context is also seen primarily as an ethical context that engages with stories lived and people's everyday life experiences, it has the potential to be therapeutic rather than as a form of social control.

Case Study

I now turn to a case study to illustrate how the use of CMM, modified to include the exploration of Quranic stories with Muslim clients, may help to produce a therapeutic intervention that is integrative of Islam and Muslim clients' belief systems. The names and some of the details of the case have been changed to ensure anonymity.

Salima referred herself to me for family therapy. She was asking for help in her relationship with her son, Shahid. She had two children, an elder daughter who was twenty-three years old and Shahid, who was twenty-one years old. The family was of Pakistani origin but the children had grown up in England. Salima and her husband had recently divorced after twenty-five years of marriage, and she described her husband as controlling and having mental health problems. The children still saw their father but had a fairly estranged relationship with him.

The particular difficulties she was having with Shahid were that he was unemployed and smoking cannabis, which she worried about, and this resulted in regular arguments between them. Shahid agreed to come and see me with his mother.

Shahid described how he was a musician and used to be a member of a band, which was doing well and about to break through to a recording contract. He admitted that he used to smoke cannabis with his friends in the band. His musical interest and lifestyle, though, were sources of huge conflict with his mother, who told him that music was *haram* (impermissible) in Islam. One day, under pressure to please his mother, he decided to quit the band. The band went on to be successful, and since then he felt depressed and had increased his cannabis smoking. For some time he didn't know what to do with himself. Eventually he developed an interest in photography and thought about pursuing a course in it. Once again, his mother told him photography was *haram*, and he relinquished his interest in it. Now he felt totally lost and spent most of his time at home, smoking cannabis regularly, and the arguments and resentment between him and his mother were growing.

I worked with Shahid and his mother together for some time on their relationship patterns and communication. We discussed the impact of the family relationships, including the separation of Shahid's mother and father and its effect on him, leaving him as the only man in the household, and the expectations that his mother had of him, as well as other matters. On some occasions, I would see Salima or Shahid separately when we thought it would be beneficial for them to have some space for themselves to explore issues, and we would then come together again for a family session to share these perspectives.

In one session with Shahid, as we discussed his future prospects, he said to me, "I will never be a good enough son for my mum unless I am willing to be sacrificed like Ismail was by Abraham." This reference to a Quranic story struck me as I had been exploring the meaning of stories in the Quran with a European Islamic scholar, Halima Krausen. One of the things I had realized in these study sessions were the many different layers of meanings within the stories and the questions they raised. So I started to explore these with Shahid through reflexive questions. I wondered what kind of a father Abraham was, what Ismail and Abraham's relationship was like, how Ismail knew that his father was acting on the command of God, and what Ismail's own relationship with God was like. I wondered if there were any other meanings in the story, other than the dominant one that Shahid had expressed, which was one of an obedient son who follows his father's and God's command. We discussed how, in the story, Abraham also had to face doubts when he was asked to sacrifice his son and struggled with the whisperings of Iblis (Satan), who appeared to him three times, attempting to deter him from what he was commanded to do.

Shahid reflected that the story may also hold the meaning of Abraham being tested to sacrifice what was most precious to him for the sake of God, possibly to detach from his son so he could be closer to God. I suggested a third possible meaning to Shahid, one that had not occurred to me but that had been put forward by the scholar with whom I was studying: that perhaps the story may also indicate that God did not require human sacrifice, as in the end God miraculously sends a ram and commands Abraham to sacrifice it in place of Ismail. This was in a time and context when human sacrifice was still practiced, and this divine intervention with Abraham brought an end to that practice. Halima had suggested to us that the pertinent question was, "What is a meaningful sacrifice?" which I put to Shahid. He began to question whether the so-called sacrifices he was making for his mother were really for her or God as they were only serving to create resentment in him toward her. This opened up conversations about whether he thought music and photography were *haram* and how he could explore if this was the case and why, so that he could take responsibility for his own choices and actions. He acknowledged that the cannabis and other drug taking was *haram* and was preventing him from moving forward in his life.

In subsequent sessions, we explored with his mother the meanings that emerged in this story and her expectations of obedience from her son. Salima acknowledged that while she thought the drug taking was no doubt *haram* and perhaps also the music and the lifestyle that went with it, she wasn't so sure about the photography. I asked Salima, was she certain she was asking Shahid to give up these things for her or for the sake of God? She realized that her attempts at controlling Shahid were because she feared losing him, as she lost her husband. She thought the drug taking was objectionable for her personally as well as Islamically. We also uncovered a deeper loss, when Salima told of how she had been separated from her own biological mother and brought up by her father and stepmother. I focused further on the impact of this on her in individual sessions. She was open to Shahid exploring with theologians the Islamic view on photography but wanted him to change his lifestyle and to stop the cannabis smoking.

Analysis

The theme of obedience featured heavily in this case. In terms of the multiple embedded levels of context and meaning outlined in the CMM model, the following analysis can be applied: Shahid's comment of "not being a good enough son unless he was willing to be sacrificed like Ismail" and the argumentative episodes with his mother can be seen in the context of their relationship in which the mother expected obedience from him in not pursuing his musical career or photography in order to be a "good son." This can be understood in the context of his individual life script where he was struggling with trying to find out his own abilities and purpose. This in turn is in the context of a complicated family script in which there is the loss of his father and thus greater expectations from Shahid to be the good son and not turn out as his father, as well as Salima's loss of her own biological mother and possible beliefs she may have held about being a "bad daughter" for having left her mother (even though in fact she was taken forcibly by her father). The fear of loss and having "to let go" featured heavily in this family's script. In the hierarchy of contexts, the theme of obedience is further compounded by the Pakistani cultural context in which hierarchical relationships between parents and children and duties and obligations to the family are heavily stressed. Add to this the religious context and the dominant cultural reading of the story of Abraham and Ismail as one of an obedient son who follows his father and God, and you have the dominant story told of how a good son is an obedient son who sacrifices his own desires.

This contextual prefigurative force downward that shapes who we are in stories told is very powerful.

Reworking the meanings in the story and exploring alternative possibilities in which it is not just Ismail who is an obedient son but also Abraham as a father who is willing to sacrifice or let go of his attachment to what is most precious to him for his relationship with God puts the ethical imperative on both children and parents in relationship. This shifts the dominant cultural script of obedience toward parents and deontic logic of duty and what ought to be to the possibility of recontextualizing both Salima's and Shahid's relationship to God. The reflexive questions generated allowed for the implicative force of stories lived or practical lived experience to become stronger rather than the contextual prefigurative forces. If God did not require human sacrifice, what would Shahid need to do to be a good enough son from God's perspective and from his mother's perspective? What would Salima need to do to be a good enough mother? It was important to recontextualize and separate out Salima's expectations from those of God. In fact, I often find in family therapy with Muslims that the parental view is projected onto God, so that it becomes a form of social control. Here, in terms of CMM, the dominant story told of obedience is a strong cultural script and was in coherence between the generations and across the multiple contexts of meaning, but Shahid's attempt to coordinate his lived experience with others was causing him distress. I hypothesized that the depression and cannabis smoking were symptomatic of this. Shahid had to find meaning in and find alternative ways of being a good son rather than doing things under the guise of obedience but harnessing resentment, and he needed to find ways of communicating this to his mother. A more conscious approach was proposed by him exploring with scholars if music and photography were really *haram*. They both had to be mindful of the other side of the story if they were to achieve coordination in CMM terminology. The management of meaning is this complex interaction in which we participate, in our attempt to fit our stories with others and our wider sociocultural and religious contexts.

I argue that exploring the religious context was vital in this case as it had the capacity to contextualize and rework long-held cultural and familial beliefs from a more ethical perspective if it was done in a way that was genuinely curious and open to mystery. Then it can call into being new meanings and creative ethical possibilities that may also develop deeper understandings of Quranic stories and people's relationship with God. Drawing on the context of religion to do this, while challenging the embedded dominant cultural stories told about obedience, kept them connected to their broader religious worldview and what they held dear. According to Cronen and Pearce (1985), CMM advocates what they call "cosmopolitan communication"—in other words, "pluralism." This enables communication with others who may have different ideas, values, and backgrounds, without one party trying to change the other. They go further in considering dialogue to be ethical communication. They also raise the question that if we contribute to one another's construction of social reality, how should we properly interact with one another? Cronen and Pearce (1985) propose that we should communicate with one another as human beings, not objects to dominate, and thereby create a better social reality. This is not only morally correct but also enables us to discover more about reality. The therapeutic context may provide a space for this discovery.

Integrating Systemic Practice and Islamic Perspectives

In the above example, I have tried to illustrate how Quranic stories can be used therapeutically to open up dialogue that can lead to learning and change.

The approach taken in this case study could be seen as top-down, bringing Islam into Western psychotherapies—in this case, systemic ideas into a modified version of CMM. But it could also be seen as bottom-up, importing Western strategies into an inherently Islamic approach, as using teaching stories, including Quranic stories, is a well-known method of transformative teaching used traditionally, for example, in the Mathnawi of Jalaluddin Rumi.

Kakar (1992) argues that myths, legends, and images can be read as a collective historical conscious. They are a rich source of psychological information and forge our collective identity. They structure our thoughts and reflections—serving to organize our inner and outer experiences and also reflect an individual's interpersonal bonds with their cultural and religious worldviews. Because the Quran features so heavily in the life of Muslims and prophetic stories are oft-repeated, it can be argued that people's internal mythology is connected to prophetic stories (Robert Abdul Hayy Darr, personal communication, November, 2017).

Bridges and Barriers to Integration

On the one hand, in its attempts to take a more holistic perspective through engaging with multiple contexts, systemic theory for me has some overlap with Islamic notions of unity in diversity, the interconnectedness of life, and the idea of monotheism: oneness—*tawhid*.

Quranic verses keep pointing to interconnectedness, turning from God to nature, to creation, to man. For example:

> Soon we will show them our signs in the furthest horizons and in their own souls, until it becomes manifest to them that this is the Truth.
>
> (41:53)

In fact, Bateson (1972), who was one of the early pioneers of systemic therapy, was a strong advocate of non-dualistic thinking. Bateson thought linear thinking was reductionist and favored a circular approach focusing on relationship, form, and pattern when working with human systems, which allows for interconnectedness and complexity as opposed to the compartmentalization so characteristic of Cartesian dualism, which not only separated mind from body but also the person from society and religion from science during the European Enlightenment. In fact, toward the end of his life, Gregory Bateson wrote a book with his daughter Mary Catherine Bateson called *Angels Fear: Towards an Epistemology of the Sacred* (1988). Despite being critical of religion and a staunch scientist, his daughter writes, "He had become aware that the unity of nature that he had affirmed in his book 'Mind and Nature' may only be comprehensible through the kind of metaphors familiar from religion; that in fact he was approaching that integrative dimension of experiences he called the 'sacred'" (Bateson & Bateson, 1988, p. 2). Furthermore, for Bateson, the subject of epistemology (the rules we use for making sense of the world) was an intensely moral concern (Hoffman, 1985). For me, these ideas fit with an Islamic metaphysical approach to science and holistic thinking in which the human being is seen as a microcosm of the macrocosm of the universe, that is, constantly interconnected with the environment and where mind, body, and spirit are interconnected in health and illness.

Systemic therapy has in practice, though, been colored by the largely Western ethnocentric cultural context in which it mainly exists. It has not been able to advance this radical thinking of Bateson's and operates in health care systems that are dominated by dualistic approaches to mind and body and the individual and society. In Krause's (2007) critique of systemic approaches to culture, she argues that systemic therapists dropped the kind of cultural complexity that was evident in Bateson's early work on the Iatmul and Naven ritual through which he tried to understand relationships and kinship structures in traditional societies. Nora Bateson (2016), the youngest daughter of Gregory Bateson, is also now trying to revive his ideas in the systemic field.

So although, in practice, systemic therapy has been beset by the Western cultural contexts in which it is practiced, through the turn to social constructionism there is some acknowledgment of this relativism. The engagement with other cultural and especially religious contexts remains superficial, with little knowledge of the actual content of diverse beliefs and different worldviews. Nonetheless, the idea of context and CMM, in theory, has presented me with the opportunity to bring the religious context into my work and to engage in a more meaningful way with it, as well as with the cultural context, and thus to understand Muslim families from a more holistic perspective and through the complex embedded contexts in which they operate.

On the other hand, the challenges some Muslims may face in working therapeutically with Quranic stories centers around issues of authority: Can they interpret meanings for themselves without relying on a scholar, and also, is it possible to accept plurality of meanings that may be derived from these stories? For Muslims, Quranic stories are the truth, and so they may struggle with the social constructionist idea of there being no single truth. Kutuzova (2010), in her paper on narrative practice and Christian beliefs, outlines similar struggles that Christians may face in the use of narrative ideas. She argues that the main difficulty that Christians who study narrative practice face is that the Christian faith means believing in the truth and distinguishing "truthfulness from falsehood." She questions whether this "questioning of truth inevitably creates doubt and destroys faith" and goes further in wondering if it is possible to acknowledge a plurality of descriptions of reality and at the same time be true to one's own inner subjective experience of truth.

This raises the question of what the truth is, or *haqq* as the Quran refers to it. Meyer et al. (2011), in their description of the ninety-nine names, point out that the word *haqq* in Arabic as a verb becomes *haqqaqa*, meaning "to journey into the heart of the night and at the same time to exert oneself to the outmost degree" (p. 58). I would argue that the psychotherapeutic process is often about such a struggle. Only by engaging with the pain and unknowing of what to do when faced with difficult relationships and with genuine human dilemmas are we called into this struggle. In my experience, in this dark struggle our faith can be tested as well as be renewed and strengthened. If we are able to respond to such situations in a truthful and balanced way, then we have the opportunity to do good and act with beauty—*ihsan*. This suggests that truth (*haqq*) may not take one form but instead require us to be in a state of openness and receptivity that can help us to understand things in a broader and more complete way, enabling us to act in truth in the best possible way we can. Halima Krausen, one of the scholars with whom I studied and from whom I learned this technique, referred to Quranic stories as "truth stories" with "moving images," again suggesting that as we engage with them, different truths may appear, and these may change depending on our state and position and who we identify with in the story. Barnet Pearce (2014), when asked in an interview if the social constructionist perspective in CMM necessitated giving up belief in a divine being or grand narrative, answered "no," but suggested we would need to look at the kind of world we create when we affirm that belief in certain ways. As a communication theorist, he said he was interested in the effect such an assertion of truth has; it does a certain kind of "work," creating certain kinds of episodes, relationships, and politics. We may want to reflect on alternatives to this approach if it does not create an ethical world. As referred to earlier, Cronen and Pearce (1985) argue that pluralistic views may indeed help us to discover more about reality. Interestingly, a hadith of the Prophet (as reported by Al-Ghazali in *The Revival of Religious Sciences*) said, "There is not a verse of the Quran that does not have an outer layer and an inner layer and not a letter, but it has a limit, and for every limit there is an expansion."

In his blog post on the nature of the Quran and its multiple levels of interpretations (*tafsir*), Michael of East Java (2015) makes the point that on the one hand the Quran is simple and accessible to everyone, and on the other it is complex and you can study it your whole life and still not know it all. He stresses that this is the nature of the Divine: He cannot be limited, and if He is infinite, then so must be his speech—that is, the Quran. Michael of East Java (2015) outlines six levels of understanding the Quran: the literal, the allegorical/metaphorical/symbolic, the comparative, the ethical, the mystical/philosophical, and the personal. This final level is subjective, and we are encouraged to read the Quran and feel like it is speaking to us and our current situation. Chapter 55, verse 2 (Surat al-Rahman) can be read as saying, "and it is He who is teaching the Quran," as opposed to "He taught the Quran" and so we are encouraged to apply it to our own lives. No doubt the themes in Quranic stories continue to apply to people's contemporary relationships and lives.

Kutuzova (2010) addresses the point of whether biblical stories have a different kind of truth from other narratives by drawing on the work of Meteyard (2009), who distinguishes between narrative therapy and narrative theology. He suggests that, for narrative theologians, not all stories have the same weight, and that there is a difference between everyday narratives and divinely inspired stories in the Bible. Idris Shah (1976) discusses the different nature of teaching stories, which he argues exist in all cultures. In a talk about learning from stories, particularly focusing on Sufi stories, he argues that teaching stories require analogical and not systematic thinking. Although they may also have cultural significance—for entertainment value or a moral lesson or to be used to reinforce a belief—what makes them distinctly teaching stories is that they are likely to be open-ended, enabling a variety of interpretations. This is because their purpose is to ultimately change the thinking process itself. They can reflect ourselves to us and our barriers to learning. They can also contain a means to self-correction through feedback. Shah (1976) suggests that once we think into them and take on different parts, we develop the capacity to be more flexible and versatile and understand more things about life and ourselves, as well as become more integrated into life and the ability to learn from it. These secondary and indirect effects are very powerful. Similarly, Robert Ornstein (2002) notes,

> On the surface, teaching stories often appear to be little more than fairy or folk tales. But they are designed to embody—in their characters, plots and imagery—patterns and relationships that nurture a part of the mind that is unreachable in more direct ways, thus increasing our understanding and breadth of vision, in addition to fostering our ability to think critically.

Shah (1976) stresses that for the Sufis, the purpose of the story is the teaching contained within it; it is therapeutic and self-educational. He distinguishes this from when stories are used for religious, didactic, and moral purposes that reinforce power systems and make people attach to the system or become dependent on the authority figure, rather than the teaching within the story. As suggested earlier, some Muslims may struggle with not submitting to authoritarian interpretations, as much of religion in the Muslim world is taught in this didactic, authoritarian way and people are discouraged from engaging with the Quran in such a way as to make their own interpretations. In fact, often people will suggest to me that therapists should seek fatwas from Islamic legal experts to instruct their clients on what would be the Islamic thing to do in a particular situation. But at a conference with legal scholars at the Centre for Islamic Legislation and Ethics (CILE), through our dialogue it became clear to me that fatwas have a role at the extremes to protect human life and dignity, but that prior to that there is much room for exploration. In fact, I would argue that Muslims are in need of these spaces for exploration, learning, and growth. Dogmatic and authoritarian approaches run the danger of taking away from our rich Islamic tradition, which in fact encourages self-exploration and understanding. The Quran again and again encourages self-reflection and self-knowledge, when, for example, it repeatedly states in chapter 13, verse 3, "For surely in this are signs for people who reflect." The Quranic premise in the stories of the prophets is that they are seeking truth, which frequently means not accepting the authoritarian dogma of their time. Irene Alexander (2008), in her book on conversations between narrative therapy and the Christian faith, also argues that if Christian counselors aspire to follow Jesus, who no doubt criticized the dominant discourses of his time, it is incumbent on them to show the same courage. I know this can be challenging; as one student commented to me, "It is hard to ask questions about these stories as they are so sacred." I would argue that if we don't question, then we idealize the prophets and we don't engage with their stories in a way that can enable us to learn about the human condition—our shortcomings and potential and, moreover, God's mercy. For surely these stories are teaching about the human struggle. For me, exploring Quranic stories has opened up new and rich meanings that, although challenging, have also deepened my faith.

Conclusion

Integrating Islam and systemic psychotherapy has no doubt enhanced my work with Muslim clients. It has improved my engagement as well as enabled me to develop techniques and interventions that are more meaningful and effective for clients. I think the therapeutic space, if it is felt to be safe and accepting, can be a mirror and really help people explore themselves as well as their relationship with a merciful God. In order for this to work, I think it is imperative that psychotherapists also study the rich traditions of Islam and explore their own relationship with God, in addition to their chosen therapeutic modality.

As I said earlier, I was fortunate to meet scholars who encouraged me to ask questions and themselves had a sophisticated understanding of human beings and their psyches. This has been invaluable for me in challenging and deepening my faith and building my own relationship with God, as well as building my confidence to address the more prevailing authoritarian approaches to Islam. Surprisingly, what I have found is that when presented with genuine human dilemmas and if people are asked questions rather than given the answers, something more ethical and beautiful can come into being, and the response is often not so black-and-white. Like anything that is cross-disciplinary, there are challenges from both sides. We need to be critical of both sides and courageous if we are going to ask the difficult questions at the interface. Bateson, in naming his final book *Angels Fear: Towards an Epistemology of the Sacred*, "advocated asking questions that disturb faith, so that the questions may define a region where angels fear to tread" (Bateson & Bateson, 1988, p. 136). He thought, "Most of the religions of the world showed little humility in their espousal of answers but great fear about the questions they will ask" (Bateson & Bateson, 1988, p. 136). Similarly, we need to hold psychotherapy to account for its lack of engagement with different worldviews and its bias toward secularism. Religion can often feed into psychopathology, but its inner spiritual dimension can also be a great source of healing and transformation. Religion and psychotherapy are both well placed to learn from one another as they deal with the human condition. In fact, the work of what we now consider psychotherapy was traditionally carried out, and still is in many places, by spiritual healers—shamans and mystics (Kakar, 1984). We should also not be afraid to borrow and integrate ideas, so long as we can root them in Islamic principles and ontology, as did the early Islamic scientists with Greek philosophy.

References

Alexander, I. (2008) Power: A conversation between narrative ideas and Christian perspectives. In I. Alexander and R. Cook (eds.), *InterWeavings: Conversations between Narrative Therapy and Christian Faith*. North Charleston, SC: Create Space Books.

Bateson, G. (1936). *Naven, a survey of the problems suggested by a composite picture of the culture of a New Guinea tribe drawn from three points of view.* Stanford, CA: Stanford University Press.

Bateson, G. (1972). *Steps to an ecology of mind.* New York: Jason Aronson.

Bateson, G. (1977). The birth of a matrix of double bind and epistemology. In M. Berger (Ed.), *Beyond the double bind.* New York: Brunner Mazel.

Bateson, G., & Bateson, M. C. (1988) *Angels fear: Towards an epistemology of the sacred.* New York: Bantam Press, p. 53.

Bateson, G., Jackson, D., Haley, J., & Weakland, J. (1956). Toward a theory of schizophrenia. *Behavioral Science, 1,* 251–264.

Bateson, N. (2016). *Small arcs of larger circles: Framing through other patterns.* Axminster, England: Triarchy Press.

Burnham, J. B. (1986) *Family Therapy.* London: Tavistock Publications.

Cronen, V. E., & Pearce, W. B. (1985). Towards an explanation of how the Milan method works. In D. Campbell & R. Draper (Eds.), *Applications of systemic therapy,*69–84. London: Grune & Stratton.

Dallos, R., & Draper, R. (2000). *An introduction to family therapy.* Buckingham: Open University Press.

Hoffman, L. (1985). Beyond power and control: Towards a "second order" family systems therapy. *Family Systems Medicine, 3*(4), pp. 381–395.

Kakar, S. (1984). *Shamans, mystics and doctors: A psychological inquiry into India and its healing traditions.* London: Allen & Irwin.

Kakar, S. (1992). *The analyst and the mystic: Psychoanalytic reflections on religion and mysticism.* Chicago: University of Chicago Press.

Khan, M. S. (1986). *Islamic medicine.* London: Routledge and Kegan.

Kleinman, A., & Good, B. (Eds.). (1985). *Culture and depression: Studies in the anthropology and cross-cultural psychiatry of affect and disorder.* Berkeley: University of California Press.

Krause, I. B. (2007). Reading Naven, towards the integration of culture in systemic therapy. *Human Systems, 18,* pp. 112–125.

Krause, I. B., & Miller, A. C. (1995). Culture and family therapy. In S. Fernando (Ed.), *Mental health in a multiethnic society: A multidisciplinary handbook. pp.* 148–171. London: Routledge.

Krause, I. B. (Ed.). (2012). *Culture and reflexivity in systemic psychotherapy.* London: Karnac.

Kutuzova, D. (2010). *Narrative practice and Christian belief.* https://dulwichcentre.com.au/explorations-2010-2-daria-kutuzova.pdf

Malik, R. (2000). Culture and emotions. In C. Squire (Ed.), *Culture and psychology,* pp. 147–62. London: Routledge.

Malik, R., Fateh, R., & Haque, R. (2009). The Marlborough Cultural Therapy Centre. In S. Fernando & F. Keating (Eds.), Mental health in a multiethnic society: A multidisciplinary handbook, 2nd ed. (pp. 174–186), London: Routledge.

Meyer , W. A., Hyde, B., Muqaddam, F., & Khan, S. (2011). *Physicians of the heart: A Sufi view of the ninety-nine names of Allah.* San Francisco: Sufi Ruhaniat International Michael of East Java (2015). *The nature of the Quran and its levels of tafsir.* https://perspectivesofafellowtraveler.wordpress.com/2015/07/10/tafsir-talk-1-the-nature-of-the-Quran-and-its-levels-of-tafsir/

Ornstein, R. (2002). *Afghan teaching stories and the brain.* Talk given at the Library of Congress, October 16, 2002. https://www.youtube.com/watch?v=hQkhijkh5Ww

Pearce, W. B. (1999). *Using coordinated management of meaning.* http://www.pearceassociates.com/essays/cmm_seminar.pdf

Pearce, W. B. (2014). On coordinated management of meaning. https://www.youtube.com/watch?v=HvME-Y5A3Og

Shah, I. (1976). *Learning from stories.* https://www.youtube.com/watch?v=ira3HsO4Yeo

Teaching Stories. https://en.wikipedia.org/wiki/Teaching_stories

Yon, K., Malik, R., Mandin, P., & Midgley, N. (2017). Challenging core cultural beliefs and maintaining the therapeutic alliance: A qualitative study. *Journal of Family Therapy.* https://onlinelibrary.wiley.com/doi/full/10.1111/1467-6427.12158

Outlining a Case Illustration of Traditional Islamically Integrated Psychotherapy (TIIP)

Hooman Keshavarzi, LPC and Fahad Khan, PsyD

ISLAM IS the second-largest religion in the world and the third-largest religion practiced in the United States (Pew, 2015). Significant research demonstrates that Muslims tend to be more reluctant to seek mental health treatment for their psychological distress relative to other groups (Sheikh & Furnham, 2000; Pilkington, Msetfi, & Watson, 2012). Among the barriers adversely impacting help-seeking behaviors among Muslims are concerns around religious, spiritual, and cultural sensitivities (Inayat, 2007; Aloud & Rathur, 2009).

Research on therapist-client matching demonstrates that similarity between therapists and their clients enhances the therapeutic alliance (Presnell, Harris, & Scogin, 2012). Though similarity provides the context for psychological growth, it is insufficient unless therapists facilitate a qualitatively new experience to help their clients better relate to their distress (Smith & Trimble, 2016). With Muslims, therapist-client matching can be at times a necessary condition, but it is not a sufficient one as Muslim clients not only need to share the same faith with their therapist but they are also likely to want their therapist to demonstrate spiritual competencies in providing a more spiritually integrated approach. In fact, it has been demonstrated that religiously oriented therapists have a significant positive impact on clients who are religiously observant (Anderson et al., 2015; Weatherhead & Diaches, 2010).

Additionally, Muslims have been shown to avoid seeking psychotherapy services if therapists are not providing it within a religious or spiritual context (Amri & Bemak, 2013; Killawi et al., 2014). Secularly oriented therapies may often offer treatments with reference to Euro-centric conceptions that are alien to the Islamic ethos or foreign to the Muslim psyche, thereby adversely rupturing the therapeutic alliance and engendering mistrust between therapist and client (Inayat, 2007). A ten-year literature review of Islamic psychotherapies highlighted the emergence of interest in this field as well as an underrepresentation of Islamic frameworks and approaches to not only provide access but also efficaciously engage Muslim mental health (Haque, Khan, Keshavarzi, & Rothman, 2016). Thus, more concrete and tangible publications are necessary to provide guidance on how to effectively integrate Islamic traditions into the psychotherapeutic encounter.

This chapter offers a case demonstration of traditional Islamically integrated psychotherapy (TIIP) originally published by Keshavarzi & Haque (2013). The Islamically integrative psychotherapeutic model is summarized briefly followed by therapeutic goals that are consistent with the framework. These therapeutic goals are qualified across sessions through a demonstration of a client suffering from social anxiety.

Traditional Islamically Integrated Psychotherapy

Although the field of psychology nourished and established itself in the West in the nineteenth century, philosophical precursors discussing human psychology were ever-present in the Muslim world as early as the ninth century (Badri, 2013; Qureshi & Rehman, 2015; Awaad & Ali, 2015, 2016). Since then, many Muslim philosophers and scholars have written on the topic. Some have highlighted psychotherapeutic frameworks as well. Keshavarzi and Haque (2013) presented an Islamically integrated psychotherapeutic framework that outlined Islamic beliefs with regard to health, pathology, human ontology, and epistemology. It also aimed to filter modern behavioral research toward an integration of psychological interventions that are consistent with Islamic principles. Ultimately in this model, health is seen on a holistic continuum that includes the acquisition of virtuous behaviors, beliefs, and spiritual practices rather than an absence of clinical pathologies.

Drawing upon Islamic belief, everyone is born on the *fitrah*—that is, a primordial, well-natured desire to connect with God that requires nurturance through appropriate socialization. The human being is ultimately responsible for aspiring to spiritual excellence, and health is achieved through the nourishment of the respective composite parts of the human psyche that permit a person to be on the pathway toward God-consciousness and actualization of one's full spiritual potential. Therefore, the ultimate goal is to attain nearness to God, whereby the lower limits of obligatory health are manifest through achieving salvation in the afterlife (Keshavarzi & Haque, 2013). In fact, if a Muslim is free of any clinical pathologies, this is not necessarily an indicator of health. Rather, the holistic refinement of the person's spiritual self leads to health. For example, an individual may not meet the threshold for narcissistic personality disorder, though narcissistic traits are very serious spiritual maladies that may potentially lead to personal and social problems in this world as well as warranting punishment in the hereafter. Therefore, narcissistic traits fall within the scope of intervention as one is to be purified from such character flaws.

Internal Framework of the Human Psyche

Keshavarzi and Haque (2013) outlined the composite parts of the human psyche as the *aql* (cognition), *nafs* (behavioral inclinations), *ruh* (spirit), and *qalb* (the heart; see Figure 7.1). The *qalb* or heart is the container for all health and pathology. Note that the term "heart" can imply the physical structure as well as its spiritual aspect. Inputs from any of the domains results in the "blackening" or conversely "radiance" of the heart (see Table 7.1).

Keshavarzi and Haque (2013) have opted to translate the *nafs* as behavioral inclinations. Its essence is not intrinsically evil; rather *nafs* reflects an automaticity of behavioral inclinations based upon its training and discipline (*tarbiyah*). In its untrained state, *nafs* is hedonistic and can be likened to Freud's conception of the id acting purely to please itself and fulfill its base carnal desires. However, through its refinement and training, *nafs* progresses through its developmental stages (*ammarah*, *lawammah*, and *mutma'innah*) and naturally inclines toward virtuous

TABLE 7.1	
Outlining the effects of the elements of the human psyche on the heart	
ELEMENTS OF HUMAN PSYCHE	**EFFECTS**

Cognition—*Aql*
 ▸ Reason
 ▸ Logic
 ▸ Thoughts
 ▸ Beliefs
 ▸ Knowledge
 ▸ Biases
	Heart—*Qalb*
	 ▸ Formation
	   of personality traits
	   • Narcissism
	   • Arrogance
	   • Jealousy
	   • Envy
	   • Deceit

Behavioral Inclination—*Nafs*
 ▸ Appetite
 ▸ Desires
 ▸ Sexual needs
	• Self-consciousness
	   • Kindness
	   • Openness
	   • Shyness
	   • Modesty

Spirit—*Ruh*
 ▸ Sensations
 ▸ Unconscious elements
   • Dreams
   • Visions
   • Catharsis
   • Sudden awareness
 ▸ Wisdom
 ▸ Purpose and meaning
	▸ Behavioral expressions
	 ▸ Effects on relationships
	 ▸ Residual effects on
	   • *Aql*
	   • *Nafs*
	   • *Ruh*
	   • *Ihsaas*

Emotion—*Ihsaas* ▸ Adaptive/maladaptive emotions ▸ Response to exogenous stimuli ▸ Endogenous emotions	

and godly behaviors. The *aql* is the rational faculty of a person. It acts purely on logic, reason, and acquired intellectual beliefs. It also determines its conclusion based on past knowledge and experiences or schemata. The *ruh* is the spirit and life force of the human being and has an affinity for the sacred, spiritual remembrance; a thirst for meaning and purpose; and a longing for the divine. All three are interconnected, and a change in any one domain will have an accompanying impact on the rest of the system (see Figure 7.1). For example, a hedonistic behavioral addiction can lead to cognitive rationalizations engendering distortions in belief and a reduction in spiritual practices, ultimately blackening the heart. We have also opted to include *ihsaas* or emotions as another domain, though previously listed under *ruh* in the original article. This is on account of significant advancements in emotion theory that may warrant an addition to the original Ghazalian conceptualization of the previously listed human domains.

FIGURE 7.1 COMPOSITE ELEMENTS OF INTERNAL HUMAN PSYCHE

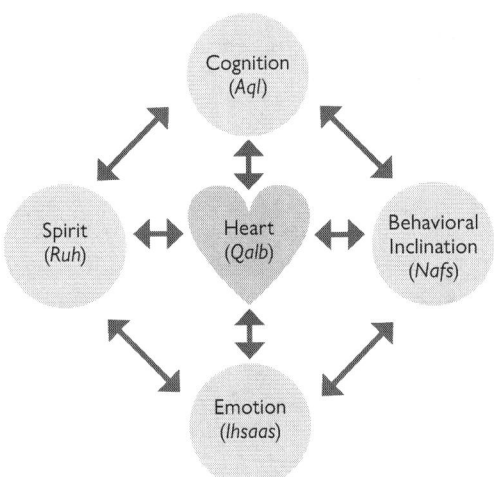

Social Contextual Framework of Existence (Ijtima'i)

Islam emphasizes a collectivistic approach to society, rather than an individualistic one. Consequentially, many Muslim cultures globally are collectivistic. Ibn Khaldun, a fourteenth-century scholar and historian, stated that "compassion and affection for one's blood relations and relatives exist in human nature as a divine gift put into the hearts of men. It makes for mutual support and aid . . ." (Rosenthal, 1969, p. 98). Ibn Khaldun considered support and harmony within a community as a central factor for its well-being and prosperity (Gierer, 2001). Modern Western societies after the Industrial Revolution have gravitated toward individualism, with the exception of the religiously devout; as Fischer (2001) put it, "Faith [spirituality] often trumps individualism" (p. 367). Though significant economic gains have been associated with individualistic quasi-free economies, there have also been associated harms to human social and psychological life. A meta-analysis concluded that cultural differences between individualism and collectivism provide an explanation for understanding the differences in human behaviors from different parts of the world (Oyserman, Coon, & Kemmelmeier, 2002). Spiritual transcendence has been shown to be negatively correlated with individualism, especially for individuals from Eastern cultures (Edara, 2016). Therefore, a comprehensive model of human psychological functioning must include a socio-contextual framework. As seen in figure 2, in this framework individuals not only focus on the internal aspects of their functioning but also keep the external systems in mind.

FIGURE 7.2. CONTEXTUAL FRAMEWORK
OF AN INDIVIDUAL'S HOLISTIC EXISTENCE

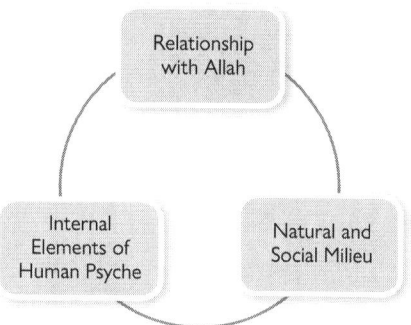

According to this framework, individuals living a holistic life focus on the internal elements of their psyche (*nafs, aql, ihsaas,* and *ruh*) coupled with their relationship with those around them as part of their spiritual growth. In the Islamic sense, individuals belong to an interconnected community and are responsible for managing their familial and social relationships, termed *huqaq al-ibad* (the rights of the servants of God). Additionally, these relationships with the environment even extend into nonhuman aspects, such as animal rights/treatment and nature. All aspects of one's internal existence are impacted by the environment. The human being is interrelational and interconnected, just as epigenetics research has demonstrated the significant impact of the environment on shaping even the brain (Roth & Sweatt, 2012). For example, development of a schema that produces automatic negative thoughts can be a result of childhood maltreatment by caregivers. Hence, one's cognitive functioning is directly affected by the context of one's environments.

Overarching Therapeutic Goals and Principles of Change

In TIIP, there are three larger overarcing goals of the psychotherapeutic encounter (see figure 7.3): *inkishaaf* (introspective self-discovery), *i'tidaal* (psycho-spiritual equilibrium), and *ittihaad* (unity of being).

Inkishaaf is an introspective self-discovery of one's current state and tendencies. In his description of achieving spiritual health, Abu Hamid Mohammed al-Ghazali, a Muslim philosopher and ascetic of the eleventh century CE, cites an Islamic tradition: "If Allah wants good for a slave, then he makes him aware of the deficiencies of his self." In fact, many Islamic scholars and historical physicians—such as Abu Bakr al-Razi, Abu Ali ibn Miskawayh, Shah Wali-Ullah, and Abu Zayd al-Balkhi—have enlisted the primacy of seeking assisted introspective awareness into one's cognitive, behavioral, and spiritual selves (Arberry, 2007; Badri, 2013; Hermansen, 1982; Keshavarzi & Haque, 2013). Awareness of self also leads to an increased relationship with God and others. Al-Ghazali cites two main modalities for achieving this aim. The first is the traditional path of Sufism, wherein one initiates oneself in a Sufi order, adopts a spiritual mentor (*murshid*), and seeks him out for assistance (Khalaf, 2014). The second modality is to find someone who can act as a process expert in human behavior and its reformation to help facilitate this introspective awareness. A modern reading of these two modalities may enlist an Islamically oriented psychotherapist as the latter process expert. One of the major goals of this therapeutic modality is to help clients engender a sense of self-awareness and understanding/conceptualization of their own cognitive, emotional, behavioral, and spiritual tendencies (*inkishaaf*).

The second major overarching goal of this therapeutic modality is *i'tidaal*, an equilibrium among all of the composite parts of the human psyche (*aql, ruh, nafs, ihsaas,* and *qalb*) and relational lives. For example, an individual who harbors excessive *khawf* (fear) may have an imbalance leading to anxiety symptoms and therefore needs the assistance of the therapist not only to gain insight but to direct the individual toward instilling more hope in God (*rajaa*) through therapeutic intervention.

All therapeutic strategies and outlines of the sessions are designed to address these two overarching goals toward engendering the third and final goal of *ittihaad* (integrative unity). The term used here intends an integration of these interconnected parts of the psyche to form a unity that works together in serving its primordial goal of connecting with God (*marifah*) and actualizing one's full spiritual potential. Through achieving this unity of being, clients also achieve a unification of their total being with the will of God, such that their actions become directed by what God desires of them. Though, it is advisable to integrate the expertise and collaboration of a traditional murshid when working on the third goal, given the heavier emphasis on spiritually oriented inter-

FIGURE 7.3. THEORETICAL PRINCIPLES OF CHANGE

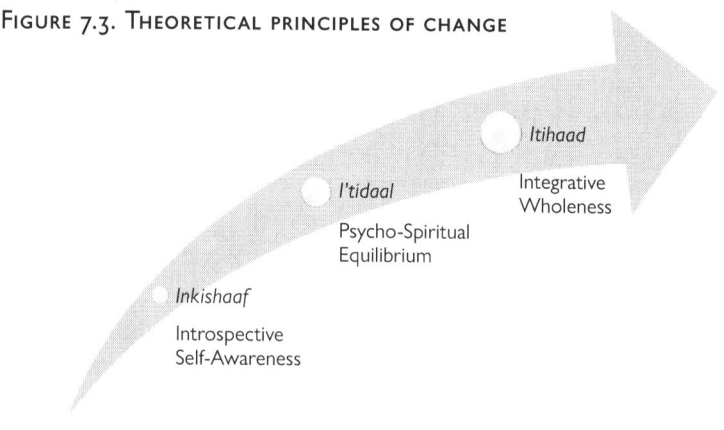

Itihaad
Integrative Wholeness

I'tidaal
Psycho-Spiritual Equilibrium

Inkishaaf
Introspective Self-Awareness

vensions. As a result of this treatment, an integrative restoring of holistic balance can provide sufficient insight into their psyche, such that they can function as their own therapists to help them when they find themselves deviating from this unity or previously achieved equilibrium.

Session-by-Session Application

In the following sections of this chapter, we describe the various sessions of therapy, followed by a demonstrated application of each group of sessions on a social anxiety case. Sessions have been grouped by assessment, identification of treatment goals, and establishment of the therapeutic alliance, then broken up by the elements of the human psyche. This Islamically integrative framework is not a strictly manualized approach, and the practitioner exercises significant flexibility, clinical intuition, and judgment. Sessional goals span several sessions, and the process of change should not be forced. A more organic and natural process of healing should be facilitated.

The following is a session-to-session demonstration of the Islamically integrated psychotherapy. The client's name and other demographic information have been changed for privacy and confidentiality purposes.

Assessment

Since the focus of the model is essentially on spiritual integration, the assessment can be divided into two components: psychiatric and spiritual, with six major goals:

- ▸ Building the therapeutic alliance
- ▸ Assessment of religiosity
- ▸ Diagnosis and conceptualization
- ▸ Assessment of internal and external psycho-spiritual functioning
- ▸ Psychoeducation and setting therapeutic goals
- ▸ Assessment of stage of change

First, it is imperative to begin the process with the primary goal of building a therapeutic alliance. Islamic spiritual writings document the salience of building trust between a spiritual practitioner and the disciple. Trust and belief in the outcome of the treatment are imperative and a necessary precondition to the practitioner working with the client. This is echoed and documented through modern behavioral research demonstrating the therapeutic alliance as being the strongest determinant variable of success in treatment. This initial phase of the therapy demands a more nondirective, person-centered approach to gathering information toward the goal of assessment and diagnosis. Person-centered interviewing strategies are recommended for gathering the typical intake data, such as the client's family, social, personal, and medical/psychiatric history (Elliott, 2004). Second, as outlined in Keshavarzi and Haque's work (2013), it is important to assess for degree of religiosity as a determinant to the degree of usage of explicit or overt mention of religious vocabulary, language, concepts, or religious references during the therapeutic encounter. The therapist must determine that the client is looking for Islamically integrated psychotherapy, and the therapist needs to provide a brief descriptor of the therapeutic orientation, style, and general outline of the therapeutic goals.

It is important to outline the conceptualization of the client's condition, revelation of the therapist's tentative diagnostic impressions, assessment of severity, etiology, prognosis, and potential therapeutic utility and outcomes of treatment. Research demonstrates that Muslims tend to prefer a more directive approach to psychotherapy (Abdullah, 2007; Dwairy, 2006; Kobeisy, 2004). Such psychoeducation generally provides the client with a greater degree of confidence in the therapist's expertise and helps set up the expectations of the therapeutic encounter. All this may not be achievable in the first session, so a working conceptualization might suffice with the intention to attain more diagnostic clarity through the course of the initial few sessions.

It is also important to assess a client's internal and external psycho-spiritual functioning using the approach outlined above. A therapist educated and trained in recognizing the functioning of the internal and external aspects of spirituality can determine its proper functioning by assessing the client's basic thought processes, emotional functioning, behavioral and instinctual inclinations, and spiritual functioning, for example—as well as a client's social functioning, including participation in the community and relationships with other individuals (relatives, community members, coworkers, etc.).

After a discussion of the therapist's preliminary conceptualization and psychoeducation regarding the condition, the therapist and client shall collaboratively develop therapeutic goals. Muslim clients may often be unfamiliar with the structure of psychotherapy, so the therapist needs to attend to any expectancy variables that may arise or be present in the room.

A therapist must also assess the client's appropriate motivation to change. As highlighted by Prochaska and DiClemente's (1983) model of change, a person who is not considering or is ambivalent about change is not likely to respond well to therapy, especially to a directive stance from the therapist. Additionally, Muslims show significant stigma and barriers for seeking treatment, and ensuring the motivation of the client is important to secure treatment compliance and commitment. A client's mere presence and reaching out may not be a good indication of level of motivation, as many Muslims may simply have been referred by clergy or family but still be significantly reluctant to engage in therapy.

To assess the client's religiosity, the therapist can administer a measure of religiosity. Although there are many such measures, we recommend using the Psychological Measure of Islamic Religiousness (PMIR) or Muslim Experiential Religiousness (MER). PMIR and MER are administered as indicators of religious growth. By administering Islamically integrated psychotherapy, it is assumed that subscales of PMIR and MER will change, thereby having a residual impact on psychological adjustment and wellness (Abu-Raiya et al., 2008; Ghorbani et al., 2016).

Case Illustration

Client Background History

Kareem is an unmarried South Asian American Muslim working professional in his mid-twenties who sought out therapy services at an Islamically oriented counseling center. He specifically requested a Muslim psychotherapist and verbalized his desire to work with his social anxiety through an Islamic framework. Kareem had struggled with social anxiety since high school. He reported living in a predominately white Christian suburb where he was bullied by his peers and struggled to fit in socially. These experiences made him very self-conscious of his behaviors, and he reported internalizing a lower self-worth during this time. Additionally, he mentioned that he grew up in a household where his father displayed significant anxieties particularly around his work, career, and finances. Kareem also has a younger sibling who struggles significantly with mental illness, and Kareem assumes a responsibility of being fully functional as a way of not placing burdens on his family.

Kareem met the diagnostic criteria for Social Anxiety Disorder. Kareem stated that he displays cognitive ruminations regarding his behaviors, becomes very distressed particularly when spontaneously asked to perform in work settings, and has fears of negative social evaluation especially in perceived high-stakes settings. This anxiety impacts his performance, causes him to become physiologically aroused, and consumes a significant amount of available cognitive resources to manage the task at hand. He has significant anticipatory anxiety and tends to practice or rehearse normative social interactions in his mind prior to his social encounters.

Forming the Therapeutic Alliance and Specification of Treatment Goals

These sessions focus on expanding the therapeutic alliance and specifying treatment goals collaboratively with the client. According to the theoretical presuppositions of motivational interviewing, individuals are unlikely to be open to change or clinical suggestions until an empathic therapeutic alliance is established (Cheng, 2007). This alliance is engendered by helping clients uncover their own discrepancies and incongruences between desired outcomes or their ideal selves and their current behaviors. This session affords an opportunity for the therapist to attain a richer understanding and appreciation of the client's summative experiences. If sufficient therapeutic alliance is not established, other treatment goals should be halted until this goal is met. At the same time, the therapist should work together with the client using a coconstructive approach in empathically following the client to identify emergent themes as they arise through empathic exploration. When determining the goals, therapists must take into account psychological, spiritual, and social functioning. The idea of balance (*i'tidaal*) must also be taken into account when determining the goals.

CASE ILLUSTRATION

The therapist utilized a person-centered approach and empathic relationship-building strategies, such as the use of open-ended questions, empathic reflections, exploratory questions, summaries of his experiences, and probing of intake questions designed to uncover patient history. The client reported feeling like a social outcast during high school. He often felt that he needed to be someone who was likeable or accepted by his peers. He talked about feeling like he was "on camera" or imagined social settings as though they were recorded interviews. This would lead to a lot of anticipatory anxiety in social settings as well as excessive anxiety and ruminative thoughts in the moment that included mind reading, where he would imagine through a negative attributive lens that his peers were poorly evaluating him in their minds. This would cause cognitive interferences, limiting his ability to be present in the moment. Upon completion of his social interactions, he would do a mental reexamination of his behaviors and others' responses and would catastrophize the perceived social errors he made. Kareem reported that his desired personality inclinations are often contingent upon what others want of him, and he harbors many "should" statements of his behaviors contingent upon his social relationships. The therapist mentally noted that at the core of his beliefs were feelings of inherent worthlessness, leading to Kareem feeling unmeritorious of social attention or connection—hence his constant attempt to perform well in social interactions in order to avoid social rejection or other potential adverse consequences, such as negative or dismissive evaluation of his worth or his fears of being fired, left jobless, and isolated. These reported experiences cause him to feel overwhelmed by his negative ruminative thoughts, intensify his feelings of anxiety, and increase his *nafsani* or behavioral inclinations of either avoidance or excessive preparation in almost scripted interactions. Ultimately, this has led Kareem to feel exhausted, hopeless, and worthless, particularly when he perceives social interactions to have gone poorly. This also caused him to decline spiritually, with diversion of focus from self-care, congruence, and God-consciousness. Furthermore, these experiences had an adverse impact on his motivation to validate his spiritual worth.

After uncovering diagnostic markers of social anxiety and affirming this diagnosis, the therapist proceeded to synthesize the client's reported experiences/symptoms in the form of the therapist's conceptualization and diagnostic impressions and used "fit" questions to gauge whether the client believed that he accurately understood his experience (Elliott, 2004). Upon affirmation of this, the therapist proceeded to share more of his conceptualization of the client's social anxiety, with a particular emphasis on the manifestation of his excessive focus on evaluation of self by others as an indicator of his own insecurities regarding his worth.

Given the client's request for Islamically oriented psychotherapy, the therapist took the liberty to explain his tentative formulation within the Islamic context of the domains of the human psyche. He illustrated this through use of a diagram displaying the interconnections of the elements of the human psyche. The therapist conjectured that the origins of Kareem's behaviors on account of his early socialization had led to some internalization of imbalanced states across the domains. These internalized cognitions have engendered cognitive distortions that shape his cognitive interpretations of events, impacting his *aql*. This then influences his *nafs*, through behaviors that produce the inclinations or compulsions to overcompensate, perform, and prepare for social settings or avoidance behaviors designed to extinguish his exaggerated activation of his emotion of fear (*khawf*). Adverse effects on his *ruh* (spirit) result, causing an over exhaustion and negligence of spiritual rituals and practices. This cycle overall leads to the manifestation of disorder localized in the heart. This vicious cycle has maintained his social anxiety. The therapist elicited client feedback at this point. The client affirmed the conceptualization.

The therapist outlined the goals for actively working to uncover factors that contribute to the maintenance of this cycle across the human elements in order to achieve *inkishaaf* (introspective self-awareness) and suggested ways of working actively to address these through the course of therapy to produce balance (*it'daal*) across all domains of the human psyche. The therapist went on to assess Kareem's motivation for change and desire to work actively both within and outside of the therapeutic setting to address his psychological distress. The client demonstrated significant relief at the therapist's tentative formulation, verbalizing a sense of assurance he felt upon having a better understanding of his suffering. The therapist's outlining of a therapeutic strategy to address this conceptualization generated excitement in the client to begin the therapeutic process.

While this previous session was a process-oriented approach to assessment, a follow-up session was conducted in order to focus on specifying the overall treatment goals based upon traditional IIP in application to Kareem's particular social anxiety. In this session, the client was oriented to a more specific explanation of the different parts of the human psyche. A diagram was drawn where the client and therapist identified activating situations and drew a circle with all the different composite parts. The therapist talked about the interconnectedness of the system and the therapeutic goal of breaking this cycle by intervening throughout the sessions on each of the systems. He also talked about cognitions, cognitive distortions, negative attribution bias, the role of religious and spiritual framing, and seeing the world through a God-centric lens. This included an evaluation of personal worth and social situations that are consistent with Islamic belief (*aqeedah*). The role of emotions was discussed, with a particular focus on emotions being a gift and avenue of connecting with God. The hadith of "ask your heart" was cited and offered a view of emotions as indicators of what behaviors should be taken. The value of bottom-up processing was discussed and how insight alone is not sufficient for therapeutic change (Elliott, 2004). An experiential unfolding and re-experiencing of emotions is necessary to facilitate change that can help rewire the currently paired episodic memories and the maladaptive shame that emerges across interpersonal situations. The *ruhani* (spiritual self) was discussed, with a focus on how the soul strives for the divine and how neglect of this system can lead to adverse psychological states. Energizing this state can provide spiritual momentum and reinforce the holistic Islamic outlook, serving as additional cues to maintaining a God-centric holistic outlook on the human experience. The *nafs* was discussed in more detail, providing the client with a horse analogy of needing to train its wild nature to become subservient to the self and the developmental stages of the *nafs*. The concept of *tahdheeb al-nafs* (refinement of behavior) was presented, with an explanation that the developmental growth of the *nafs* can be achieved through *mukhalafat al-nafs*, or opposing the unhealthy self-destructive behavioral patterns of avoidance, short-term pleasure seeking, and evasion of discomfort. Etiology was revisited and a brief discussion took place of psychopharmacology as a means of monitoring symptoms in the event that medications became warranted.

TABLE 7.2: *Treatment plan using traditional Islamically integrated psychotherapy (TIIP) model*

ELEMENT OF THE PSYCHE	TREATMENT GOALS SPECIFIC TO THE ELEMENT OF THE PSYCHE
Aqlani: Cognitive	1. Shift toward a positive attribution bias—balancing fear (*khawf*) with hope (*rajaa*) 2. Differentiation of personality (*shakhsiyyah*) from character attributes (*akhlaq*) 3. *Tawakkul:* seeing behaviors as a manifestation of God's perfect will and ultimate plan for the client 4. Letting go of control over things that can't be controlled 5. Utilizing God-centric evaluations of one's social conduct 6. Internalization of positive opposite beliefs, such as possessing inherent worth in belonging to the children of Adam 7. Challenging cognitive distortions of mind reading, catastrophizing, and shoulds 8. Embracing errors and personal acceptance in challenging perfectionism or desire to script behaviors 9. Uncovering one's avoidance hierarchy toward *inkishaaf*
Ihsaas: Emotional	1. Trusting one's emotions as indicators of spiritual directions 2. Increase emotional awareness and symbolization of salient experiences

Ihsaas: Emotional (continued)	3. Personal stories related to emotional functioning
	4. Expressing emotion
	5. Enhancing emotional regulation
	6. Actively reflecting on positive and negative emotions
	7. Making sense of experience: disembedding; creation of new meaning; insight; seeing patterns, understanding in a new way; new narrative construction
	8. Change emotion with new interpersonal experience: new lived experience with another provides a corrective emotional experience; disconfirms pathogenic beliefs; provides interpersonal soothing; new success experience changes emotion
	9. Change emotion with emotion: an alternate self-organization, set of emotion-schematic memories, or "voices" in the personality based on primary emotions are accessed by (a) attentional reallocation, (b) focus on a new need/goal, or (c) changing interactions. The maladaptive emotional response is synthesized with, or transformed by, more adaptive emotional response.
Nafsani: Behavioral inclinations	1. Mukhalafatu al-nafs al-ammarah: opposing the unhealthy self-destructive behavioral patterns of avoidance, short-term pleasure seeking, and avoidance of discomfort
	2. Out-of-session exposure to socially anxiety-provoking stimuli
	3. Embracing and confronting avoidance behaviors
	4. In-session exposure to role playing through unscripted replications of potential high-stakes social interactions
Ruhani: Soul-related	1. Muraqabah: Islamic contemplative exercises
	2. Dhikr: remembrance of God
	3. Hajj/*Umrah*: religious pilgrimage
	4. Spiritual mentorship
	5. Regular *salat*: five prayers on a daily basis
	6. Prescribed *duas* or prayers with a concentration on the meanings that challenge the faulty cognitions
Ijtima'i: Social/ environmental	1. Improvement of relationships with relatives: parents, spouse, children, siblings, extended family
	2. Greater integration of social supports in belonging and greater involvement in the community
	3. Overall care and commitment to the universality of human beings

Ruhani Health: Spiritual Interventions

These sessions may be conducted prior to cognitive, behavioral, or emotional work in the interest of generating spiritual momentum and facilitating a reconnection to Allah that can serve as a positive motivator and have a residual impact on the client's experiential and feeling states. This session is designed to evoke a primacy of purposeful spiritual connection to Allah and focus attention on nurturing one's relationship with Allah. The focus of this session is to provide psychoeducation regarding the spirit and the accompanying role of *dhikr* in nourishing the spirit. Therapists may include that the spirit is the vehicle and the life force of the human being, requiring nourishment and desiring a connection to its primordial state of being connected to Allah. A simple bifurcation of the human being into physical and spiritual being may be presented to the client. In that, the physical being was created from the earth and needs created materials to survive, such as food and clothing, whereby the soul cannot be satiated through such earthly things and was breathed into the body by Allah and has a longing for the Divine. A reference to two Quranic verses (39:22; 13:28) can be used toward this aim. These Quranic verses highlight the spiritual light or radiance (*nur*) being bestowed upon individuals blessed with complete connection to Islam and the tranquility being achieved through *dhikr* (remembrance of Allah). Conversely, the absence of the remembrance of God causes a hardening of the heart. Hardened hearts may sense a feeling of a void—an experience of a mechanistic and meaningless existence. A prophetic tradition can be used to engender motivation to a more experiential and spiritual approach to their lives. This prophetic tradition states, "Be mindful of the foresight of the believer, for verily he sees with the light (*nur*) of God." The significance of *nur* is reaffirmed in this prophetic statement demonstrating the necessity of *dhikr* to enlighten the heart with this spiritual radiance in order to provide clarity and spiritual insights into the examination of their lives that foreshadow the cognitive, emotional, and behavioral development and aspects of the psychotherapy to follow.

During this session, it is useful to incorporate some experiential healing modalities into the psychotherapy encounter. Such prescriptive techniques can be taught in session, and additional prayers and litanies can be prescribed for usage outside of the session. The *kitab al-adhkar* of Imam al-Nawawi is a recommended resource to find various prayers to be incorporated into sessions. It is encouraged that therapists gain some orientation either through an experienced Islamically integrative therapist or a spiritual healer in finding Islamic spiritual exercises to use in the therapy encounter.

CASE ILLUSTRATION

The client had been researching and looking into formal Islamic spirituality (*tasawwuf*) and was considering adopting the *naqshabandi* spiritual order. He wanted to use some therapy time to explore this possibility. The client had initiated contact with a spiritual mentor (*murshid*) and felt comfortable with him. He had informed this mentor of his work with his spiritually integrated psychotherapist and felt that the *murshid* seemed interested in a collaborative approach to helping him nurture his overall psychological and spiritual growth. The therapist in the session used empathic following and exploration to help him arrive at a conclusion as to whether he wanted to use a formal approach to spirituality or more of a personalized one. He decided that he would formally join the *naqshabandi* order and discussed with his therapist the prescription of *muraqabah* that he was given as a regimen for fifteen minutes a day. The therapist was encouraging use of this prescription and recommended diaphragmatic breathing coupled with breathing the name "Allah" in and exhaling *hu*. The therapist initiated this in the session by having Kareem close his eyes and focus on his heart. He asked him to imagine, with each breath, light originating from the heavens entering his heart and cleansing him of his anxieties, worries, and concerns and to focus on generating a trust in God (*tawakkul*), with each breath expanding the light in his chest and with each exhale a cleansing or removal of his negative energies. The client tried this in the session a couple of times and reported feeling soothed and tranquil. The therapist prescribed this to the client as a way to self-soothe whenever he felt anxious.

HOOMAN KESHAVARZI, LPC AND FAHAD KHAN, PSYD

Ihsaasi Health: Traditional Islamically Integrated Emotion-Focused Psychotherapy

These sessions largely utilize emotion-focused psychotherapy, and the research finds that the addition of emotion, rooted in emotion-focused therapy (EFT) built on dialectical constructivism, integrates well into the Islamically integrative framework (Elliott, 2004). The aim of these sessions is to help facilitate a deeper, more meaningful, and experiential processing of psychological themes with a focus on emotions. EFT focuses on the necessity for emotional accessing, symbolizing, and replacement of maladaptive or imbalanced emotion schemes through the experiential unfolding and replacement with more adaptive or balanced emotions that are better suited to meet its needs. The emergent new themes are seen as a tendency for individuals to move toward integration and reconciliation, and the therapist and client co-construct the new themes as they naturally emerge and gravitate toward growth.

Though EFT largely conceptualizes emotion through an evolutionary approach to survival, TIIP looks at emotional processing and its underlying needs as a spiritual reaching out or internal mechanism of regulation toward *i'tidaal* designed to facilitate the psychological health necessary to serve God. The difference between this TIIP conceptualization in contrast to normative EFT conceptualizations is in the form of a focus on a spiritual or religious context within emotional processing, as opposed to a more secular processing of emotional meaning. Uniquely, EFT therapists highlight emotional transformation as occurring through either replacing a maladaptive or secondary emotion with a more adaptive one or a change of maladaptive emotions through new interpersonal experiences akin to cognitive behavioral therapy (CBT)–exposure psychotherapies. The most significant technique used to facilitate such a change is through chair work that targets unfinished business with an individual (family member) or a self-critic / self-self / self-other issue. From an Islamic perspective, the self-critic has a term—*al-waidhu* (the warner)—which serves as the moral compass put in the heart of all Muslims or perhaps the *nafs al-lawammah* (the blaming self). The blaming self has a function of attempting to manage the *nafs al-ammarah bi-su*, the hedonistic lower self. Consistent with traditional Islamically integrated theory, *i'tidaal* is desired. Therefore, an overactive *nafs al-lawammah* can lead to its maladaptive expression in the form of social anxiety and production of maladaptive shame. However, the *nafs al-lawammah* can become quieted down if it begins to trust that the *nafs* is disciplined and is sincere in its desire to serve God. When such an integration between the self and *nafs al-lawammah* is achieved, a person can enter into a state of *nafs al-mutmainnah*, or contentment, whereby the *nafs al-lawammah* is more of a guide rather than a harsh critic of its internal behaviors. As seen in figure 7.4, EFT chair work can be used here to help facilitate a discussion between the *nafs al-lawammah* and the self. Thus, in these two sessions, deeper emotional processing is facilitated through use of EFT techniques that may result in emergent markers that warrant chair work. This is a more bottom-up processing technique whereby the emotions are activated in the room, and a deeper sense of change can occur through a repairing of new adaptive emotions in the moment.

CASE ILLUSTRATION

Over the course of two sessions, Kareem talked about his interpersonal challenges, particularly in the workplace, where he experienced difficulty quieting his ruminative thoughts filled with fears of failure and incompetence. This was a task marker for the therapist identifying the self-critic or *nafs al-lawammah*. The therapist set up the chair task and elicited his willingness to participate in the chairwork. The client was open to it, and the therapist asked that his internal self-critic be put in the other chair. Through this processing, his self-critic emerged as a vicious bully or the internalized voices of others containing self-defeat, beliefs of worthlessness, and incompetence. The therapist used heightening to empower and encourage the negative critic to dismiss and belittle himself. The therapist then switched them over and elicited the emotional experience of hearing such harsh self-critique. The client expressed sadness, hurt, and shame. Through a process of switching between chairs, the client started displaying assertive anger toward the *nafs al-lawammah*,

Figure 7.4 Two-chair process of addressing the self-critic in TIIP

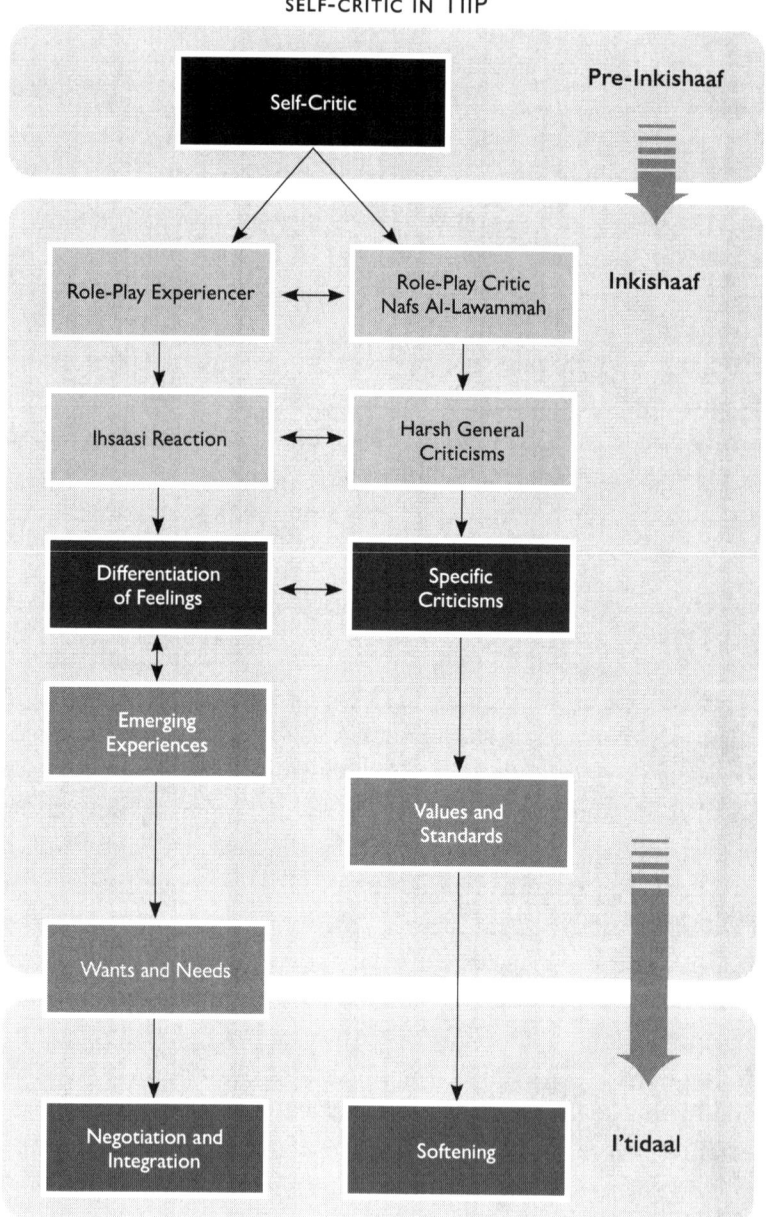

whereby the *nafs al-lawammah* began to soften. Ultimately, a unification between them emerged where the self would consider and satisify the *nafs al-lawammah*'s desire for him to excel and strive for meaning and perfection, though the *nafs al-lawammah* would ease up and allow more trust and room for himself to succeed in achievement. It was uncovered that the *naf al-lawammah*'s rigidity would lead to self-defeat and a low-ered likelihood of achievement—for example, debilitating anxiety in the face of interpersonal tasks that was nonfunctional. Thereby, through the transformative process of bottom-up processing, he was able to replace shame with assertive anger, which facilitated a balance of power. This allowed for the maladaptive shaming of the *nafs al-lawammah* to play a more adaptive function of serving the role of keeping alert and ensuring that he is adequately tuning into his moral compass.

Aqlani Health: Cognitive Psychotherapy within an Islamic Context

These sessions focus more on cognitive processes. As Keshavarzi & Haque (2013) discuss, many early Islamic scholars have written about the importance and role of cognition and thinking processes that influ-ence the remaining elements of self and ultimately induce distress and dysfunction. It should be noted that the distinction between a pure CBT approach and Islamically integrated psychotherapy is that dys-functional thinking is indicated or defined by Islamic theology and creed as opposed to the *Diagnostic and Statistical Manual of Mental Disorders* (American Psychiatric Association, 2013). For example, clients who may harbor adaptive beliefs in the form of a strong internal locus of control—sometimes a predictor of psychological well-being (Chimezie, Chibuike, & Emmanuel, 2017; Klonowicz, 2001)—may still display an imbalanced overreliance on self as opposed to giving up control to God. Though there is significant research to indicate that the secondary benefit of a balanced locus of control is better (Shepherd et al., 2006), the clinician's focus is not necessarily solely on symptom relief but rather a rectifica-tion of Islamic psychological processing that has direct primary spiritual worth or benefits and a secondary positive impact on mental health.

Thus, the client is being directed by a cognitive focusing on the role of God in his or her life and the integration of core Islamic beliefs, such as the role of trusting God (*tawakkul*), framing and acceptance of hardship and challenges as indicators of spiritual elevation (*ibtilaa*), and recognizing the role of self and the inclusion of a God-centered processing of life's circumstances whether clinical or otherwise (*muhasaabah*). Research supports the positive impact of positive religiously oriented cognitive processing as an indicator of psychological well-being and alleviation of anxiety and depressive feelings (Hodge, 2006). These sessions shall include some psychoeducation regarding the role of cognition.

Imam al-Ghazali gives the example of the *aql* or cognition as needing to be the master over the other elements because of the fact that the *aql* impacts and influences perception and plays a significant role in the interpretation of events. Additionally, individuals process meaning through the cognitive lens in which they view the world. Having a healthy understanding of Islamic theology and its application to one's personal life can help provide a positive religious framing of one's experiences (Hamdan, 2008). In emotion-focused therapy, there is more of a bottom-up processing of events, whereby during these sessions a top-down processing of the clients' experience will help to address their challenges from both angles. Though emotion-focused therapies ultimately contribute to cognitive changes as well (Elliott, 2004), these sessions are designed to have a more explicit focus on cognitive processing.

During this session, psychoeducation can be offered regarding the rational emotive behavior therapy's ABCs, where an Activating event leads to the triggering of an underlying Belief that causes a Consequence (Ellis & Dryden, 1987). Consequently, the client will emotionally experience the residual impact of his or her cognitive interpretations. CBT funneling tactics can be used to help arrive at the client's core beliefs. The diagram of situation, automatic thoughts, intermediate thoughts, core beliefs, and outcome can be illustrated by inputting the client's expressed content into the outlined process diagram. A review of the client's most commonly held cognitive distortions can be discussed as well as their impact on the human experience. The diagram can be collaboratively filled in with the client. Cognitive restructuring can also be discussed with a particular emphasis on *tawakkul* (trust of God); *ibtilaa*, or acceptance and positive framing of struggle; *rida bi-l Qadaa* (contentment with the decrees of God); *shukr* (gratitude exercises); and a God-centered interpretive frame to the client's specific life circumstances.

CASE ILLUSTRATION

As outlined above, the focus of the next sessions is on cognition. The therapist provided some psychoeducation on the role of the *aql* and cognition. He went on to illustrate the ABCs and requested that he and the client diagram his cognitive patterns and cycle. The therapist began by asking about an antecedent. The client described one activating trigger as being at work and spontaneously asked to provide a presentation of his current output. This triggers in him the automatic thoughts of, " Uh-oh. This is going to be hard. You are not prepared. People are going to be watching you." This leads him to intermediate or conditional thoughts of, "If you fail, people will think you are incompetent. You don't know what you are doing or talking about. You look foolish." His core beliefs are, "You are worthless and incompetent, and no one will want to be around you if you display your true self."

The therapist worked with the client to highlight this and focused on how he felt watching this diagram. He stated that he felt relieved to see it outlined and that just thinking that way in the moment also induced sadness and shame in him. The therapist cited the prophetic narration where God says, "I am according to the way that my slave perceives me," and talked about how our thoughts are consequential to our spiritual, cognitive, emotional, and behavioral selves. Additionally, the therapist talked about how it was not only permissible but encouraged to take a good omen (*ta'ful*), that is, being attuned to any environmental triggers to engender optimism and a more positive attribution bias about the future. Doing so with the negative is Islamically prohibited. This influences one to act more congruently with optimism, which propels positive behaviors and from a spiritual perspective attracts the spiritual radiance of God onto the circumstance/event.

The therapist and the client together uncovered his tendency to use the cognitive distortions of mind reading, fortune telling, all-or-nothing thinking, castastrophizing, and "should" statements to maintain his symptoms. The therapist asked him to try to fill this out for other situations as homework. Additionally, the therapist and the client worked together to start to identify a stronger religious lens and spiritual cognitive orientation. They were able to look at the concept of *tawakkul*, or trusting God in application to his life. He started to identify that if he were to see all events as being in the hands of a beneficent, good, and merciful Lord that knows what is best for him, he could begin to let go of control. He is able to see his imperfections as not necessarily imperfections but rather divine indications or will propelling him toward the "good" of which he may not be aware. Even a mistake by him can be seen as an expression of the perfect will of God. Rather than resisting this or attempting to take control, he is able to frame challenges as divine leadings on his pathway toward God. He may not be able to perceive the good immediately but has trust in God (*tawakkul*) that whatever outcome ensues, it is God's desire. The client identified that his job would be to do his due diligence to prepare but then resign the outcome of events to God Almighty and as outside his scope of abilities.

Nafsani Interventions: Behavioral Interventions

This domain contains perhaps the most literature in the traditional writings of Islamic spiritual practitioners. This is referred to as *tahdheeb al-nafs*, or disciplining the *nafs*. For example, Imam al-Ghazali discussed modalities of training the *nafs* in his *Ihya Uloom al-din*. Keshavarzi and Haque (2013) cited Ghazali's horse analogy and how the *nafs* requires discipline. This entails that the client embrace the discomfort in the process of rectification and reformation of the *nafs*. CBT avoidance hierarchy diagrams or charts can be useful to help outline the avoidance of discomfort that reinforces the vicious cycle of providing temporary relief albeit long-term dysfunction. Through a process of training one's behaviors, discipline is engendered and the discomfort of habituating to new behavioral patterns becomes alleviated over time. These two sessions focus on the specific behavioral tendencies that maintain the client's suffering. In the case of Kareem, his avoidance was manifested by his attempts to avoid any instances where he may be seen as unprepared, incompetent, socially awkward, or undesirable. Although, in the above sessions, the client was able to cognitively restructure his thinking, this could only translate into new habituated behaviors through exposure. Additionally, exposure response interventions can provide new corrective experiences that help to rewire the pathological connections in the limbic system that maintain the anxiety. New interpersonal experiences can permit a transformation of maladaptive anxiety with new, more positive emotions. Exposure strategies that can be utilized during the course of subsequent sessions include both in-session exposures through role play or imaginal exposures, as well as an examination of avoidance behaviors outside of the session in the client's environment.

CASE ILLUSTRATION

During these sessions, the therapist introduced the idea of working on the *nafs* or one's behavioral inclinations and the necessity, through exposure, of engendering new behaviors that disrupt the vicious cycle created by avoidances. The therapist cited the cognitive interventions conducted in previous sessions and a new necessity to translate such new insights into one's environment. The therapist discussed the necessity of embracing the discomfort and working through exposures to engender new behaviors that would, over time, become less anxiety provoking. The client expressed his motivation to begin this process. The therapist suggested that they come up with a scenario that may seem particularly anxiety provoking to him. The client stated that when he spontaneously has to present some of his work to his colleagues, this causes him intense anxiety, and he will take time to try to overly prepare, which often does not help lessen the anxiety. The therapist suggested that they role play this scenario, where the therapist can be the employer and the client would present his most recent projects to the therapist. The client seemed a little anxious but agreed. The therapist started by helping the client use his imagination to attempt to re-create the work environment in his mind. The therapist encouraged that he also verbalize his negative automatic thoughts and emotions that occurred during the course of the role play. The therapist attempted to create some spontaneity in the role by asking him various questions about the project. The therapist and client processed his experience after the session. The client stated that this was useful and talked about how he was surprised how it mirrored his actual experiences. The client reported feeling slightly more confident and wanted to try to do this in his life. The therapist asked the client to do the following homework: create a list of his avoidance hierarchy and list next to the avoidances on a scale of one to ten his level of anxiety regarding such circumstances.

The therapist and client together reviewed his avoidance hierarchy. The therapist asked the client to select which of his behaviors he would like to attempt to reform in his environment. The client selected his tendency to appear competent at all times. The therapist and client came up with exposure strategies to try to evoke his anxiety in the interest of creating corrective experiences. The therapist and client agreed upon his verbalizing to the employer when he did not know something or felt that a task was challenging. For example, he might say, "Certainly this job seems like a challenge and I may not know exactly how to tackle it right now, but I am sure I can put my effort and energies toward accomplishing this task." The therapist and client worked out a few more examples of exposures that he could implement in his environment. The therapist encouraged the client to continue to monitor his behavioral inclinations and tendencies toward avoidance of healthy alternatives to his pathological cycles. The therapist also talked about expanding this beyond his social anxiety to his overall religious activities and life, whereby he could look at his spiritual inventory and monitor whether he is able to maintain consistency on his spiritual devotions.

Conclusions

The goal of this chapter was to offer a case demonstration across sessions of TIIP, as originally published by Keshavarzi and Haque (2013). Secularly oriented therapies may often offer treatments based on Western conceptions that can be considered incongruent with Islamic philosophy or foreign to the Muslim psyche, thereby negatively impacting the therapeutic alliance and engendering mistrust between therapist and client (Inayat, 2007).

Although this was an illustration of a case of a Muslim client suffering from Social Anxiety Disorder, the basic conceptual framework rooted in the three principles of change can be generalized to other conditions. This approach is also very flexible, given its integrative orientation, permitting the adoption and adaptation of mainstream psychotherapies within the basic objectives and tenants of TIIP. When working with other conditions, the conceptualization and goals should be oriented to addressing the specific manifestations of that disorder. Given the theological or pastoral element of this model, it can be adapted for pastoral settings and for Islamic chaplains to use in the context of clinical pastoral care. Additionally, it is ideal for therapists using this approach to have a basic familiarity with Islamic theology and Muslim mental health.

Lastly, a holistic approach to psychotherapy that takes into consideration both the internal workings of the human psyche and the effects of the person's relationship with his or her physical and social milieu is recommended.

Recommendations

As recommended by Haque et al. (2016), theoretical models that are built from the philosophy of Islamic thought and within the Islamic tradition need to be expanded. Specifically, toward the end of expanding this specific theoretical orientation labeled TIIP, further exploration into the Islamic tradition is needed, with further attention to the Sufi literature informing additional practical interventions that can be adopted within its framework. Such literature mining may focus on the *tahdheeb al-nafs* (behavioral reformation) and *tadheeb al-akhlaq* (character formation) writings, given their convergence with the subject matter of psychology. Islamic contemplative exercises such as *muraqabah* (discussed above) or cognitive strategies outlined in the books of Islamic spiritual practitioners have tremendous potential to be implemented in practice. Finally, after an identification and integration of various treatment methodologies within this framework, outcome studies need to demonstrate the utility of these interventions to particular sets of problems in order to validate the efficacy of such interventions.

Aql	Nafs	Ihsaas	Ruh
Table 7.3. *Maladaptive manifestations across domains*			
"I am incompetent." "I look goofy." "I'll probably mess up."	Avoidance behaviors	Secondary fear, maladaptive shame	Spiritually depleted; exhaustion and fatigue
"What people think of me is important." "If I do not perform well, people will not like me." "If I am not interesting, people will not want to be around me." "If I do not perform well, people will see my deficiencies and fire me."	The desire to please others Pre-scripted practice of interactions	Emotional dependence on others	Intentional incongruence with religion
"I believe I am worthless, incompetent, and unlikable." Fear of abandonment Worthlessness/weakness	Overly critical self	Lack of emotional intelligence and dysregulation	Religious despondency

References

Abdullah, S. (2007). Islam and counseling: Models of practice in Muslim commu-
nal life. *Journal of Pastoral Counseling, 42*, 42-55.

Abu-Raiya, H., Pargament, K. I., Mahoney, A., & Stein, C. (2008). A psychological
measure of Islam religiousness: Development and evidence for reliability and
va- lidity. *International Journal for the Psychology of Religion, 18*(4), 291–315.

Aoud, N., & Rathur, A. (2009). Mental health and psychological services among
Arab Muslim populations. *Journal of Muslim Mental Health, 4*, 79–103.

American Psychiatric Association. (2013). *Diagnostic and statistical manual of mental
disorders* (5th ed.). Arlington, VA: American Psychiatric Publishing.

Amri, S., & Bemak, F. (2013). Mental health help-seeking behaviors of Muslim
immigrants in the United States: Overcoming social stigma and cultural mistrust. *Journal of Muslim Mental Health, 7*(1), 43–63.

Anderson, N., Heywood-Everett, S., Siddiqi, N., Wright, J., Meredith, J., & McMillan, D. (2015). Faith-adapted psychological therapies for depression and anxiety: Systematic review and meta-analysis. *Journal of Affective Disorders, 176*,
183–196.

Arberry, A. J. (1979). Sufism: An account of the mystics in Islam. New York: Harper
& Row.

Arberry, A. J. (2007). *Razi's traditional psychology*. Damascus, Syria: Kazi
Publications.

Awaad, R., & Ali, S. (2015). Obsessional disorders in al-Balkhi's 9th-century
treatise: Sustenance of the body and soul. *Journal of Affective Disorders, 180*,
185–189. doi:10.1016/j.jad.2015.03.003

Awaad, R., & Ali, S. (2016). A modern conceptualization of phobia in al-Balkhi's
9th-century treatise: Sustenance of the body and soul. *Journal of Anxiety Disorders, 37*, 89–93. doi:10.1016/ j.janxdis.2015.11.003

Badri, M. (2013). *Translation and annotation of Abu Zayd al-Balkhi's* sustenance of
the soul. Richmond, VA: International Institute of Islamic Thought.

Cheng, M. S. (2007). New approaches for creating the therapeutic alliance:
Solution-focused interviewing, motivational interviewing, and the medication
interest model. *Psychiatric Clinics of North America, 30*(2), 157–166.

Chimezie, N., Chibuike, O., & Emmanuel, K. (2017). Role of locus of control and
gender on psychological well-being among youth athletes. *Journal of Psychology
and Sociological Studies, 1*(1), 177–185.

Dwairy, M. (2006). *Counseling and psychotherapy with Arabs and Muslims*. New
York, NY: Teachers College Press.

Edara, I. R. (2016). Relation of individualism-collectivism and ethnic identity to
spiritual transcendence among European Americans, Asian Indian Americans,
and Chinese Americans. *Counseling and Values, 61*, 44–63.

Elliott, R. (2004). *Learning emotion-focused therapy: The process-experiential approach to change.* Washington, DC: American Psychological Association.

Ellis, A., & Dryden, W. (1987). *The practice of rationale-emotive therapy.* New York: Springer.

Fischer, C. S. (2008). Paradoxes of American individualism. *Sociological Forum, 23,* 363–372.

Ghorbani, N., Watson, P. J., Madani, M. & Chen, Z. J. (2016). Muslim Experiential religiousness: Spirituality relationships with psychological and religious adjustment in Iran. *Journal of Spirituality in Mental Health, 18*(4), 300–315.

Gierer, A. (2001). Ibn Khaldun on Solidarity ("Asabiya")—Modern science on cooperativeness and demand empathy: A comparison. *Philosophia Naturalis, 38,* 91–104.

Hamdan, A. (2008). Cognitive restructuring: An Islamic perspective. *Journal of Muslim Mental Health, 3*(1), 99–116. http://dx.doi.org/10.1080/15564900802035268

Haque, A., Khan, F., Keshavarzi, H. & Rothman, A. E. (2016). Integrating Islamic traditions in modern psychology: Research trends in last ten years. *Journal of Muslim Mental Health, 10*(1), 75-100.

Hermansen, M. K. (1982). Shah Wali Allah's arrangement of the subtle spiritual centers. *Studies in Islam,* 137–150.

Hodge, D. R. (2006). Spiritually modified cognitive therapy: A review of the literature. *Social Work, 51,* 157-166.

Inayat, Q. (2007). Islamophobia and the therapeutic dialogue: Some reflections. *Counseling Psychology Quarterly, 20,* 287–293.

Keshavarzi, H., & Haque, A. (2013). Outlining a psychotherapy model for enhancing Muslim mental health within an Islamic context. *International Journal for the Psychology of Religion, 23*(3), 230–249.

Khalaf, M. (2014). *Mukhtasar Ihya ulum ad-din* (A. Ghazali). Lypia/Nikosia, Cyprus: Spohr. Publishers.

Killawi, A., Daneshpour, M., Elmi, A., Dadras, I., & Hamid, H. (2014). *Recommendations for promoting healthy marriages & preventing divorce in the American Muslim community.* http://www.ispu.org/pdfs/ISPU_Promoting_Healthy_Marriages_and_Preventing_Divorce_in_the_American_Muslim_Community.pdf

Klonowicz, T. (2001). Discontented people: Reactivity and locus of control as determinants of subjective subjective well-being. *European Journal of Personality, 15,* 29–47.

Kobeisy, A. N. (2004). Counseling American Muslims: Understanding the faith and helping the people. Westport, CT: Praeger.

Oyserman, D., Coon, H. M., & Kemmelmeier, M. (2002). Rethinking individualism and collectivism: Evaluation of theoretical assumptions and meta-analyses. *Psychological Bulletin, 128,* 3–72.

Pew Research Center. (2015, May 12). *America's changing religious landscape.* http://www.pewforum.org/2015/05/12/americas-changing-religious-landscape/

Pilkington, A., Msetfi, R. M., & Watson, R. (2012). Factors affecting intention to access psychological services amongst British Muslims of South Asian origin. *Mental Health, Religion & Culture, 15*(1), 1–22.

Podikunju-Hussain, S. (2006). *Working with Muslims: Perspectives and suggestions for counseling.* http://www.counseling.org/knowledge-center/vistas

Presnelli, A., Harris, G., & Scogin, F. (2012). Therapist and client race/ethnicity match: An examination of treatment outcome and process with rural older adults in the Deep South. *Psychotherapy Research, 22*(4), 458–463.

Prochaska, J., & DiClemente, C. (1983). Stages and processes of self-change of smoking: Towards an an integrated model of change. *Journal of Consulting Clinical Psychology, 51,* 390–395.

Qureshi, R. K., & Rehman, Q.H. A. (2015). Islam and human psychology. *Pakistan Journal of Commeerce and Social Sciences, 9*(3), 1012–1016.

Rosenthal, F. (1969). *Ibn Khaldun, the muqadimah.* Bollinger Series, N. J. Davord (Ed.). Princeton, NJ: Princeton University Press.

Roth, T. L., & Sweatt, J. D. (2012). Epigenetic mechanisms and environmental shaping of the brain during sensitive periods of development. *Journal of Child Psychological Psychiatry, 52*(4), 398–408.

Sheikh, S., & Furnham, A. (2000). A cross-cultural study of mental health beliefs and attitudes towards seeking help. *Social Psychiatry and Psychiatric Epidemiology, 35,* 326–334.

Shepherd, S., Owen, D., Fitch, T. J., & Marshall, J. L. (2006). Locus of control and academic achievement achievement in high school students. *Sage Journals, 98*(2), 318–322.

Smith, T., & Trimble, J. (2016). *Foundations of multicultural psychology: Research to inform effective practice.* Washington, DC: American Psychological Association.

Swift, J., Greenberg, R., Whipple, J., & Kominiak, N. (2012). Practice recommendations for reducing premature termination in therapy. *Professional Psychology: Research and Practice, 43,* 379–387.

Vidair, H. B., Feyijinmi, G. O., & Feindler, E. L. (2017). Termination in cognitive behavioral therapy with children, adolescents, and parents. *Psychotherapy, 54* (1), 15–21.

Weatherhead S. & Daiches, A. (2010). Muslim views on mental health and psychotherapy. *Psychology and Psychotherapy Theory: Research and Practice.* 75–89.

CHAPTER 8

Marrying Islamic Principles with Western Psychotherapy for Children and Adolescents

SUCCESSES AND CHALLENGES

Fyeqa Sheikh, PsyD

ISLAM AND PSYCHOLOGY are typically seen as two opposing disciplines, given the cultural stigma associated with mental health. However, an Islamic understanding of personality and psychopathology has been present for centuries. Currently, given the anti-Muslim sentiment in the United States, the need for mental health services among the Muslim community is paramount. With increased awareness of mental health issues and services has come a rise in use of mental health services. Therefore, it is essential that the psychological community at large understand how Islamic principles can be incorporated into Western psychotherapy. Researchers have outlined strategies to incorporate Islamic values into psychotherapy with adults (Abu-Raiya & Pargament, 2010; Abu-Raiya, 2015), yet there is a paucity of research concerning utilizing Islamic psychology principles with children and adolescents.

Adolescence is a time period that is culturally bound. In the United States, legal markers define the end of adolescence; one is seen as an adult at the age of eighteen. In other cultures, however, the time of adolescence is seen as a more fluid concept and is defined by traditional rites of passage such as marriage. Adolescence is a time when an individual is exploring his or her values and identity formation is occurring. It is historically seen as a time of storm and stress as well as conflict with parents. Often this conflict occurs regarding values and is accentuated when there is a difference in religious values between parents and their children. A therapist's task is often to find middle ground between the parent and child dyad.

Children, on the other hand, filter information through their parents and other adults; thus, the influential adults in their lives shape their religious values. A child's understanding of religious mores and values is contingent upon his or her developmental and cognitive level. For instance, a child who is in the preoperational stage of development according to Piaget (1936) might see religion as black or white, with little room for a gray area, whereas a child who is in the formal operational stage may be able to abstractly reason and interpret information in a more complex manner to form his or her own opinion.

Parents attempt to educate their children on Islamic values based on their own upbringings and how they make sense of their own Islamic identities. In collectivistic cultures, grandparents and other extended family members are also responsible for passing on cultural and religious values. Parents may also enroll their children in full-time or weekend religious education courses to augment their child's learning. As the child matures, peers may also influence one's values. Specifically in the teenage years, peers often become more influential than parents in terms of one's likes and dislikes. This can also extend to one's understanding of right and wrong.

Given the importance of the family system in the Islamic tradition, where the needs of the family are often prioritized over the needs of the individual (Hodge, 2002; Ali, Lieu, & Humedian, 2004; Smither & Korsandi, 2009; Weatherhead & Daiches, 2015), it is only natural that therapy with children and adolescents involve the entire family system. Including the family system in psychotherapy can be beneficial, while also presenting key challenges. In this chapter I discuss my integration of Islamic principles into Western psychotherapy with children, adolescents, and families and how I navigate potential challenges in engaging with this population. Further, I will discuss challenges and recommendations for creating a framework for Islamic psychotherapy.

Islam

It is estimated from research conducted in 2015 that there are approximately 3.3 million Muslims in the United States, which accounts for approximately 1 percent of the total population (Mohamed, 2016). Islam is a monotheistic religion that began in the seventh century with the words of the Quran being sent to the prophet Mohammed (peace be upon him; Ross-Sheriff & Husain, 2004). Muslims believe that the holy book, the Quran, is the word of Allah (God), and encompasses a complete way of life, including sociopolitical domains (Ross-Sheriff & Husain, 2004). Sharia, or Islamic law, governs many Muslim-majority countries, thus leaving little room for the separation of religion and state (Ross-Sheriff & Husain, 2004). A Muslim is one who follows the way of Islam and declares that there is no god but Allah, and Mohammed (peace be upon him) is his last and final messenger. Islam holds that Muslims must follow the right path in order to achieve a righteous and fulfilling life (Ross-Sheriff & Husain, 2004).

Five main pillars of Islam serve as the primary tenets of the faith. *Shahadah* (declaration of faith) is the first pillar and contains the only words required for an individual to become a Muslim (Al-Mateen & Afzal, 2004). *Salat* (prayer), the second pillar, requires Muslims to supplicate five times a day facing Mecca. The third pillar, *zakat*, holds that individuals distribute 2.5 percent of their savings annually to those in need. The fourth pillar, *sawm,* requires individuals to abstain from food, drink, and sexual activity from dawn to sunset in the holy month of Ramadan, which is based on the lunar calendar. The fifth pillar of Islam, *hajj,* is the annual pilgrimage to Mecca in Saudi Arabia that Muslims must complete at least once in their lifetime if they are able to financially afford it (Seda, 2002).

Beyond these basic tenets of Islam, Muslims are also prescribed lifestyle requirements to which they must adhere. These include abstaining from foods considered *haram* (forbidden) or foods that include pork or are pork-based products (Hoot, Szeci, & Moosa, 2003). Many Muslims also only eat *zabiha* (permissible) meat that is slaughtered in adherence to an Islamic method and in the name of Allah. Alcohol and any form of intoxicants are also prohibited in Islam. In terms of interpersonal relationships, there is often separation between males and females, with intermingling between the sexes not generally condoned unless it is for business or academic purposes. Furthermore, community or *ummah* holds great importance in Islam, and the religion promotes the interconnectedness of family (Pridmore & Pasha, 2004). Community prayer, *jummuah*, is conducted at the *masjid* (mosque) on Fridays, which is a holy day for Muslims.

Islamic Psychology and Psychopathology

Although authors (Ali, 1995; Abu-Raiya, 2015; Mohamed, 1986; Utz, 2011; Bonab & Kooshar, 2011; Mohamed, 1995) have attempted to discuss the intersection between Islam and psychology, at present, a unified definition of Islamic psychology does not exist. York Al-Karam (2017) discusses the lack of articulation of a unified definition of Islamic psychology with reference to previous authors who have contributed to the field. She conceptualizes the discipline of Islamic psychology through the multilevel interdisciplinary paradigm as "the interdisciplinary space where psychology, subdisciplines, and/or related disciplines engage scientifically about a particular topic and at a particular level with various Islamic sects, sources, sciences, and/or schools of thought using a variety of methodological tools" (York Al-Karam, 2017, p. 4). Drawing on the definition York Al-Karam proposed, for the purposes of this chapter, *Islamic psychology* refers to an understanding of human nature and the psyche based on the early work of Muslim scholars and philosophers and how that interplays with Western psychology and psychotherapy.

Psychology in Arabic is referred to as *ilm-al-nafs* (science of the self). According to Al-Ghazali (1058–1111), one of the most revered early scholars of Islam and who wrote on human nature, he argued that the self or psyche (*nafs*) comprises various states: *nafs-al-ammarah* (the ordering self), which is seen as the most unhealthy and egotistical; *nafs al-lawwama* (the blaming and evaluating self); and *nafs al-mutmainna* (the calm and peaceful self; Ali, 1995; Husain, 2006). The term *nafs* is sometimes used interchangeably with *ruh* (soul), which also encompasses drives, feelings, thoughts, behaviors, and will (Husain, 2006). The *ruh*, also referred to as the "spirit of man" (Keshavarzi & Haque, 2013, p. 239) either drives a person away from the will of Allah or closer to him (Ali, 1995). Through the use of *aql* or *ilm* (intellect and knowledge) the individual is able to differentiate between good and evil and direct his or her behavior toward the will of Allah (swt). It is posited that human behavior is driven by *fitrah* or the innate tendency to believe in the oneness of Allah (*tawhid*) and worship Him (Khalil et al., 2002). Despite the innate tendency toward goodness, environmental forces may allow one to turn away from the will of Allah (Mohamed, 1995). Further it is understood that cognition occurs not only within the brain but also within the *qalb* (heart). The *qalb* is essential for following the path of Allah. The *qalb* is also highlighted as the source of spiritual disease and unrest (Husain, 2006). Muslim scholars (e.g., Al-Ghazali) differentiate between the physical body and the spiritual self (Ali, 1995). The physical body is composed of flesh, whereas the spiritual aspect of the self is the essence of man, and the heart is the center (Ali, 1995).

Psychopathology, according to Islamic scholars, emerges from an imbalance between the worldly and spiritual needs (Khalil et al., 2002). Al-Ghazali also viewed psychological illness as resulting from spiritual distance from Allah. Diseases that originate in the *qalb* may also bring about psychopathology, including envy, ignorance, cowardice, cruelty, lust, doubt, malevolence, deception, and greed, as these conditions are viewed as deviations from the will of Allah (Husain, 2006). According to Al-Ghazali, these diseases or blemishes are a result of the evil propensity of the *nafs*, dormancy of the *aql*, or lack of good reason (Keshavarzi & Haque, 2013). Another origin of psychopathology may be experiencing religion as restrictive or negative (Murken & Shah, 2002). Furthermore, misusing the freedom and choice given by Allah (swt) can result in undesired symptoms (Sheikh & Gatrad, 2000). Essentially, from an Islamic psychology perspective, the features of the self are in conflict and must be balanced in order to achieve a well-adjusted sense of self. The goal of Islamic psychology is to have the *nafs* attain unconditional tranquility (*nafs al-mutmainna*) while the sick psyche is referred to as *nafs-al-marid'a* (Abu-Raiya, 2015). It involves regulating one's behavior in the direction of Allah's will and attaining both worldly and spiritual success. In an Islamic psychology perceptive, the Quran and hadith (written collection of sayings and actions [S] of the Prophet Mohammed [peace be upon him]) set bounds and limits, and the goal is to help individuals return to the straight path (Inayat, 2005).

Cognitive Behavioral Therapy and Systemic Approach

Cognitive behavioral therapy (CBT) is a Western-developed therapeutic approach that posits that thoughts or beliefs, emotions, and behaviors are interrelated. It holds that the way an individual interprets a situation affects how he or she feels and acts. Through CBT, cognitive errors (errors in the way of a person's thinking) are identified. Further, maladaptive thoughts are challenged and reframed, and replaced with more adaptive thoughts and behaviors. Key strategies in CBT include building a collaborative relationship between the therapist and the client, a general agenda set by the clinician, Socratic questioning, homework, and cognitive restructuring (Pearce et al., 2015).

When working with children and adolescents, one must also consider the individual's context. Uri Bronfenbrenner's (1977) ecological systems theory posits that an individual interacts with four ecological systems that affect his or her development. These include the microsystem, which encompasses the individual's immediate surroundings, including relationships with parents as well as one's school; the mesosystem, which refers to the interactions between the individuals who make up the mesosystem, such as the interaction between an individual's parents and the school; the exosystem, which corresponds to factors that are impacting the child indirectly, such as a life event occurring for the parent; and the macrosystem, referring to cultural and societal beliefs, including religion (Bronfenbrenner, 1977). CBT and ecological systems theory function in harmony, due to the importance placed on context in CBT.

Congruence and Conflict of CBT and Ecological Systems Theory with Islam

Saunders, Miller, and Bright (2010) have identified that in Western-oriented psychotherapy, clinicians' approaches fall on the spectrum of avoiding the client's spiritual and religious beliefs and practices (SRBP) to engaging in spiritually directed care. Avoiding a client's spiritual beliefs can be a careless practice, due to lack of acknowledgment of the association between spiritual, physical, and mental health (Saunders et al., 2010) as well as neglecting to address a dimension that may be playing a significant role in the client's life. Assessment of the importance of one's spiritual beliefs and connection is essential to determining the role that spirituality will hold in psychotherapy. Researchers (Abu-Raiya & Pargament, 2010) have identified that Islam is central to the lives of Muslims, so psychotherapists should ask about religious beliefs when working with Muslim clients. Furthermore, Islam is a multidimensional construct; thus, it is paramount that the clinician assess one's degree of religiosity and spirituality when working with a Muslim client. During the intake, when I am gathering information about the client's background and history, I also assess any cultural and spiritual beliefs that are important to the client. Many times throughout my clinical practice, a client has sought me out as a clinician due to my faith background. Particularly when working with children and adolescents, it is often important to the parents that the clinician share the same faith background due to concern about how the clinician's understanding of Islam may impact treatment as well as concerns about how differing values may impact rapport.

This was the case with my work with Sarah, an eight-year-old Muslim girl who presented to therapy due to obsessive thoughts that were sexual in nature and corresponding guilt after being exposed to sexually graphic content by a peer. (All names and personal details of clients described in the manuscript have been modified to maintain anonymity.) It was of utmost importance to the parents that the clinician shared the Islamic faith due to fears that a therapist approaching their daughter from a Western perspective may not fully understand Sarah's guilt and the taboo around illicit sexual content from an Islamic perspective. Sarah's case is discussed further in this chapter as a means of conceptualizing the utilization of a CBT, a systemic, and an integrated Islamic psychology approach.

Islamic psychology is often viewed in contrast to Western psychology due to the criticism that Western psychology rationalizes guilt and prefers individualistic goals (Jafari, 1993). While this may be largely true, especially in the case of CBT, other aspects of CBT are congruent with psychotherapy in an Islamic context. Beshai, Clark, and Dobson (2013) have identified points of conflict between Islam and CBT as well as how CBT can be adapted to fit one's religious values. According to the authors, Islam is more rationalistic than constructivistic (i.e., an absolute reality exists) while CBT is constructivistic (i.e., reality is constructed). In Islam, there are absolute truths and "should" statements (e.g., one should pray five times a day), while in CBT, "should" statements are avoided (Beshai, Clark et al., 2013). Furthermore, there may be issues with hypothesis testing as some issues may be viewed as concretely wrong in Islam, such as homosexuality or consuming alcohol. Thus, attempting to rationalize a client's guilt about consuming alcohol can be counterproductive. It can also be difficult to change core maladaptive schemas that are rooted in Islamic values. In Islam, it is believed that all positive events as well as all adversities originate from Allah, so Muslim clients may believe that they do not have control over their circumstances. (Islam stresses the notion that humans possess free will and must take responsibility for their actions. Some individuals, however, may interpret predetermination as lack of control over their lives.) This is in contrast to CBT, which aims to empower the individual by reinforcing the idea that he or she has control over his or her environment, thinking, and behavior (Beshai et al., 2013).

Despite these points of conflict, CBT can be congruent within an Islamic framework with certain modifications. Religiously integrated CBT has proven to be effective in reducing clients' symptoms of anxiety (Vahidid-Motlagh & Kajbaf, 2011) and depression (Pearce et al., 2015). Furthermore, Pakistani students viewed many aspects of CBT congruent with Islamic principles (Naeem et al., 2009). CBT statements can be modified to fit one's religious values (Beshai et al., 2013; Hodge & Nadir, 2008). Hodge and Nadir (2008) provide examples of how traditional CBT statements can be modified in an Islamic perspective. For instance, the statement "Because I often make myself undisciplined and self-defeating by demanding that I absolutely must have immediate gratification, I can give up my short-range 'needs'—look for the pleasure of today and tomorrow—and seek life satisfaction in a disciplined way" (Hodge & Nadir, 2008, p. 34) can be modified to "Allah (God) gave us free will, including the ability to control our *nafs* (self). In addition, Allah has also given us many opportunities to practice self-control through fasting during Ramadan and weekly Sunna (traditional) fasting on Mondays and Thursdays. These are ways, with the help of Allah, we can enhance our self-discipline and change for the better" (Hodge & Nadir, 2008, p. 37). My work with Sarah helps demonstrate how to use a more flexible approach when working within a CBT and systemic context.

Sarah

As stated earlier, Sarah is an eight-year-old Muslim girl who presented to therapy due to obsessive thoughts that were sexual in nature and guilt after being exposed to sexual content by a peer. Sarah's guilt was impacting her ability to sleep, eat, and socialize at school. She also refused to attend school and faced issues separating from her mother. Given her close relationship with and dependency on her mother, Sarah's compulsion took the form of an overwhelming need to relay every minor transgression to her mother to attain relief from her anxiety. Furthermore, she experienced extreme guilt in regard to seemingly minor transgressions (e.g., having a negative thought about someone). Sarah's parents considered themselves moderately religious. Sarah attained her religious education from Sunday school as well as through the influence of immediate and extended family.

From a traditional CBT standpoint, Sarah's guilt would be rationalized through cognitive restructuring (e.g., "There is nothing wrong with having sexual thoughts. Sexual thoughts are a normal part of life."). The therapist may also utilize exposure techniques by exposing Sarah to her sexual thoughts, which, given Sarah's understanding of sexual relations in Islam, may promote additional guilt. These actions would be counterproductive as they are attacking core beliefs that are rooted in Islamic principles.

Within a combined CBT, systemic, and Islamic psychology context, I stressed the importance of *qadr* (divine will) and that Sarah did not necessarily possess agency in having these thoughts appear. Addressing the case from a systemic perspective, it was also essential to involve Sarah's parents in treatment. Sarah's father was not available for psychotherapy sessions due to his work schedule, but her mother was an active member of therapy; a portion of each session was devoted to meeting with her individually or with Sarah present in the room. Sarah's mother was encouraged to provide education on the Islamic stance on sexual relations between men and women. It was discovered through the therapy process that Sarah's mother, while trying to protect her daughter and proceeding with the best intentions, would enable Sarah's behavior by allowing her to stay home from school. Sarah's mother also provided reassurance when Sarah would confess her sins, which, in fact, reinforced Sarah's anxiety. Sarah's refusal to attend school was handled in a manner that is consistent with behavioral therapy (i.e., not enabling the refusal and dropping Sarah off at school every day). It proved essential to involve the school, a significant aspect of Sarah's microsystem. Her school counselor was involved in the treatment, and consultation with her allowed Sarah to have a place in school to seek refuge when she experienced difficulties managing her anxiety. The school counselor and I collaborated closely (as part of the mesosystem) to ensure that there was continuity of treatment goals in both settings. Sarah's mother was also advised not to submit to reassurance-seeking behavior, which is known as *response prevention*. Sarah's symptoms can be conceptualized through an Islamic psychology lens, as her *nafs-al-lawwama* (the aspect of the self that promotes guilt) is in overdrive, promoting excessive guilt. From an Islamic psychology standpoint, psychopathology can also be seen in her case as emerging from viewing religion as restrictive or negative.

According to researchers (Abu-Raiya & Pargament, 2010; Beshai et al., 2013), religion, namely Islam, can be a means of coping. Clients can choose how they want to interpret certain Islamic principles, such as the belief that adversity comes from Allah. Such beliefs may promote feelings of learned helplessness as clients feel that they may not have control over their circumstances (Beshai et al., 2013). On the other hand, an individual may view religion as a means of coping leading to positive health effects (Beshai et al., 2013). In Sarah's situation, religious principles were utilized as a means of managing anxiety brought on by response prevention techniques and obsessions. A fundamental component of CBT is differentiating between a thought and a behavior. This idea was instrumental in helping Sarah experience her thoughts as *just* thoughts. I reinforced the notion that Sarah was not acting on her thoughts. Further, the concept of intention (*niyya*) in Islam is cornerstone, as intention is viewed at times (depending on the school of thought) as more important than action. *Niyya* is regarded as the aspect that provides importance to one's action (Qara'ati, 2014). If an action is conducted without intention, or with evil intention, it is deemed invalid (Qara'ati, 2014). Each act of worship that is conducted should be conducted for the pleasure of Allah rather than worldly recognition, praise, or reward (Qara'ati, 2014). This concept can be extrapolated to thought; although a thought may be negative (e.g., sexual thoughts that are unprovoked), there is no ill intention and no action on these thoughts. Therefore, I encouraged Sarah to understand that it is not her *niyya* to have these sexual thoughts, which proved to be beneficial in reducing her feelings of guilt.

The use of specific techniques to aid Sarah in better managing her anxiety also proved to be effective as practiced in traditional CBT. Third-wave CBT has incorporated the use of mindfulness techniques to help the individual be more conscious in the present moment (Brown & Ryan, 2003) as well as to disavow the power of thoughts. *Salah* (prayer) in Islam can be seen as a form of mindfulness in which an individual is attempting to focus his or her attention solely on the actions of *salah* rather than other worldly matters. *Salah* reduces psychological distress, keeps structure and discipline, offers strength in times of hardship, and allows individuals to express their feelings, hopes, and needs (Ashy,

1999). *Salah* was prescribed to Sarah as a means of positive coping and dealing with anxiety in conjunction with traditional mindfulness techniques. Rather than journaling, which is often prescribed in traditional CBT, Sarah was asked to speak directly to Allah and perform *dua* (supplication) to improve well-being.

It is also essential to take into account Sarah's developmental and cognitive level in her understanding of Islamic principles. According to Piaget (1936), Sarah is in the concrete operational stage of development, allowing her to demonstrate concrete reasoning and possess understanding that her thoughts and feelings may not be shared by others and may not be part of reality. Given Sarah's tendency to think in concrete terms, her understanding of Islam was based on absolute right and wrong rather than room for interpretation and gray area. This tendency impacted the therapeutic process as elder extended family members and teachers at Sunday school often told Sarah that thoughts and intentions should both be pure. This notion also contributed to increased distress for Sarah, especially when she had a thought, for example, that her cousin looked ugly. She experienced extreme guilt and felt compelled to confess her thoughts to her mother to assuage her guilt and anxiety. Encouraging Sarah to ask for *tawbah* (repentance) regarding these thoughts proved to be productive in reducing her anxiety, while also reminding her that she does not will her thoughts to appear as mentioned above.

Saima

The concept of *qadr* (divine will) was discussed previously and, as noted by Beshai et al. (2013), can be used by clients as a means of learned helplessness and rejecting change strategies. As witnessed in my clinical work, the concept of *qadr* can be reframed to help clients view their circumstances as originating from Allah rather than of their own doing. Saima, an adolescent who was diagnosed with a chronic health issue, demonstrated the tendency to be self-critical and self-blaming when it came to this issue. She believed that her actions had caused the illness or that Allah was punishing her by diagnosing her with this condition.

Utilizing the cognitive strategy of reframing, I helped Saima understand that her actions did not cause her illness and that she was not personally responsible for these circumstances. The concept of all events, positive and negative, originating from Allah helped Saima cope with her illness. It was also reinforced that her illness was a test that was provided to her by Allah. Furthermore, utilization of Quranic verses such as "Indeed with hardship comes ease" (94:6) and "On no soul doth Allah place a burden greater than it can bear" (2:286) instilled hope in Saima.

Challenges from an Islamic Perspective in Engaging with Children and Adolescents

When working with families within the Islamic and psychological domains, many challenges may present themselves. Being a practicing Muslim myself, I am often concerned about imparting my own values onto the client. It is essential that the therapist be aware of his or her own biases when working within a religious context and attempt to approach the client from an unbiased standpoint. I strive to approach each case through an unbiased lens and am transparent with my clients about my faith background. Furthermore, I am not an Imam or scholar, and at times I worry about the depth of my own understanding of Islamic principles. To remedy this issue, I attempt to collaborate with Imams and other spiritual advisers to ensure that, when I am outside of my scope in terms of religious understanding, I can refer the client. I actively engage in research and continuing education to ensure that I am expanding my knowledge of both Islam and psychology.

A unique challenge that presents itself when engaging therapeutically with teenagers is often the difference in values between the parent and child. This leads to the struggle in identifying who the client is that the clinician is serving. When working within a systemic context, the child and the caregivers are seen as the client, but this can also extend to siblings. In my work with adolescents, I have found it helpful to work with the individual as well as one or, ideally, both parents in treatment.

HANA

Hana's case is exemplary in navigating differences in treatment goals and values in the parent-child dyad. Hana, a seventeen-year-old Muslim girl, presented to psychotherapy due to feelings of depression and depersonalization. Hana was in her junior year of high school and was struggling with increased peer pressure, lack of diversity and affiliation with peers in her school, and feeling isolated from other Muslims. Hana's mother described the family as religious, indicating that the family prays five times a day. Further, both Hana and her mother wear *hijab* (head covering). Hana has two younger brothers with whom she has a conflictual relationship. She described a positive relationship with her father but stated that he recently has been disappointed in her actions (e.g., engaging in "inappropriate" conversations with friends through social media). Hana described a more distant relationship with her mother, whom she described as "overbearing" and less forgiving than her father.

When asked about goals for therapy and primary issues that both Hana and her mother would like to address, Hana's mother discussed Hana's lack of adherence to Islamic practices such as *salah*. I met individually with Hana, and upon exploration of her values, discovered that she does indeed ascribe to the values that Islam preaches but has become less involved with ritualistic aspects of Islam including *salah*, due to her perceived inability to fully focus on this activity. She expressed a desire to return to her prayers, but found her mother's goal of praying five times a day far too unattainable. It proved important to meet with Hana's mother to discuss the idea that Hana's beliefs and values may be different from her mother's and to help her mother accept Hana's current exploration of values. The importance of allowing Hana to socialize with peers, specifically Muslim peers, was stressed to Hana's mother as well. I also met with Hana and her mother together in session to identify middle ground in Hana's mother's expectations of Hana and Hana's goals for her own behavior. I helped Hana and her mother identify a reasonable goal of adhering to prayer (i.e., once a day) and building on this goal for the future. Although I helped Hana and her mother arrive at a compromise, it is important to note that I did not suggest nor condone the idea of praying fewer than five times a day. Ideally, in retrospect, I would refer Hana to an Imam or scholar to make a determination about the religious ethics of praying fewer than five times a day. I provided psychoeducation on mindfulness and encouraged use of mindfulness to increase focus during *salah*. In order to resolve Hana's feelings of isolation from the Muslim community, it was suggested that she join a local youth group in a mosque and attend events to feel more connected.

Naiza

Another potential challenge in working with adolescent Muslim clients is when parents neither approve of nor wish to be a part of treatment. Such was the case in psychotherapy with Naiza, a nineteen-year-old, second-generation woman. Naiza's mother strongly disapproved of psychotherapy due to the stigma associated with mental health in both her religious and cultural community. Naiza would often lie to her mother about attending psychotherapy, further promoting feelings of guilt, although she knew it was necessary to address her debilitating anxiety. Naiza often brought up points of contention between her own values (friendships with non-Muslim peers, shaking hands with men) and her mother's more "conservative" values. A major challenge in working with Naiza was not being able to engage with her mother in order to identify points of compromise. Furthermore, I also experienced guilt as a result of Naiza's decision to lie to her mother about attending psychotherapy, as respect of parents is a cornerstone in Islam and lying is a forbidden act.

In addition to the challenges described above, there are also systemic and contextual constraints that are unique to my experience. The contextual constraint of being a Muslim psychotherapist in a hospital setting is that there is no structure for implementing Islamically oriented psychotherapy. In a facility where the population served is predominantly Muslim, it may prove simpler to implement specific guidelines for engaging with Muslim clients. A setting that caters to Muslim clients may also be able to promote religious accommodations for the population served, such as implementation of a *salah* space. Furthermore, ethical issues of the degree to which religion is incorporated into psychotherapy may be of less concern in a setting catering to Muslim clients. Although I engage with many Muslim clients, I am not branded as a "Muslim psychologist." Thus, clients may feel more comfortable discussing therapy issues that are laden with Islamic context in a setting with a clinician who solely or specifically engages with Muslim clients.

Challenges and Suggestions for Creating an Islamic Psychotherapy Approach

My therapeutic approach described above is an integrative approach in which the conceptualization and treatment are based on a Western psychotherapy approach with Islamic principles integrated into the treatment. Ideally, an Islamic approach to psychotherapy would initiate from the ground up, where conceptualization and treatment would both occur through an Islamic philosophical lens. Although researchers acknowledge the incongruence of some Western models of psychotherapy with Islam and call for a model that tackles the subject from the ground up (Haque, 1998; Weatherhead & Daiches, 2015), few individuals have attempted to create a true "Islamic psychotherapy." Keshavarzi & Haque (2013) have outlined an Islamic psychotherapy approach in which intervention takes place at the three levels of the self: *nafs, ruh,* or *aql*. While Keshavarzi and Haque (2013) have conceptualized treatment from a novel Islamic lens, the therapeutic elements are based on cognitive therapy such as reframing and positive religious self-talk with the incorporation of spiritual connection. Pearce and colleagues (2015) have also outlined a framework for religious CBT, which, too, is based on existing CBT principles with the integration of religious practices and beliefs. Further, Abu-Raiya (2015) has outlined a dynamic, Quranic-based model of psychotherapy, which is based on psychodynamic theory. While these models are a step in the right direction, they have not solved the issue of primary treatment being framed in Western psychotherapy approaches.

One of the challenges of creating an Islamic psychotherapy approach is the lack of training provided in spiritual matters in Western psychology training programs. Further, the lack of analysis of the works of

Islamic scholars and philosophers accounts for only a cursory under-standing of the Islamic theory of personality. As noted above, there has been movement in conceptualizing through an Islamic psychology lens and the development of an Islamic understanding of personality. Due to the bias of receiving training from a Western perspective, however, one naturally engages in psychotherapy that is congruent with his or her own clinical experience and foundational knowledge. A personal limitation for me is not being an Islamic scholar and having my per-sonal education of Islam based on my own parents and education that I received through both parochial full-time school and Sunday school. There is a depth of knowledge that I have yet to explore when it comes to religious knowledge and interpretation. Further, knowledge from an Islamic philosophical context must be obtained in order to adequately create an intervention strategy that is rooted and contextualized from an Islamic psychology standpoint.

Future Clinical Directions

I have outlined a number of conflicts and limitations in integrating Islamic principles into psychotherapy with few suggestions of how to remedy these challenges. One of the steps I can personally take to improve my clinical practice with Muslim clients is to incorporate a standardized measure of religious affiliation and further understanding of one's religious beliefs during intake. Another improvement would be to provide psychoeducation on the integrative Islamic psychology approach and the manner in which it will be integrated into psycho-therapy. Furthermore, my measure of clinical success has largely been based on qualitative measures and subjective self-reports of improve-ment. I can improve my practice by utilizing standardized measures of clinical efficacy to further assess treatment outcomes. Having a more direct relationship with an Imam or other religious scholar would be helpful in coordinating treatment. While I have referred individuals to a spiritual leader for consultation on matters that are outside of my scope, I do not have a direct relationship with an individual or center and have not coordinated care as often as I would like. Another venture for the future would be to provide further education and awareness to the Muslim community about mental health issues, specifically those impacting children, to increase utilization of mental health services. The increase in Muslim clients presenting to treatment would offer a larger research base as well as improve my clinical skills in integrating principles from Islam into psychotherapy. I am employed in a hospital located in a metropolitan city with a diverse population; thus, it is anticipated that there are many individuals from a Muslim faith background who are not accessing services, given the limited number of clients on my caseload who are of Muslim background. Therefore, it is essential that education be disseminated in schools and places of worship and to parenting groups about warning signs for mental health issues.

References

Abu-Raiya, H. (2014). Western psychology and Muslim psychology in dialogue: Comparison between between a Quranic theory of personality and Freud and Jung's ideas. *Journal of Religious Health, 53*, 326–328. doi: 10.1007/s10943-012-9630-9

Abu-Raiya, H. (2015). Working with religious Muslim clients: A dynamic, Quranic-based model of psychotherapy. *Spirituality in Clinical Practice, 2*(2), 120–133. http://dx.doi.org/10.1037/scp0000068

Abu-Raiya, H., & Pargament, K .I. (2010). Religiously integrated psychotherapy with Muslim clients: From research to practice. *Professional Psychology: Research and Practice, 41*(2), 181–188. https://doi.org/10.1037/a0017988

Ahmed, S., & Reddy, L. A. (2007). Understanding the mental health needs of American Muslims: Recommendations and considerations for practice. *Journal of Multicultural Counseling and Development, 34*(4), 207–218

Ali, A. H. (1995). The nature of human disposition: Al-Ghazali's contribution to an Islamic concept concept of personality. *Intellectual Discourse, 3*(1), 51–64.

Ali, S. R., Liu, W. M., & Humedian, M. (2004). Islam 101: Understanding the religion and therapy implications. *Professional Psychology: Research and Practice, 35*(6), 635–642.

Al-Mateen, C. S., & Afzal, A. (2004). The Muslim child, adolescent, and family. *Child and Adolescent Psychiatric Clinics of North America, 13*(1), 183–200. *Journal of Religion and Health, 38*(3), 241–257.

Beshai, S., Clark, C. M., & Dobson, K. S. (2013). Conceptual and pragmatic considerations in the use of cognitive-behavioral therapy with Muslim clients. *Cognitive Therapy and Research, 37,* 197–206. https://doi.org/10.1007/s10608-012-9450-y

Bonab, B. G., & Kooshar, A. A. H. (2011). Reliance on God as a core construct of Islamic psychology. *Social and Behavioral Sciences, 30,* 216–220.

Bronfenbrenner, U. (1977). Toward an experimental ecology of human development. *American Psychologist, 32*(7), 513–531.

Brown, K. W., & Ryan, R. M. (2003). The benefits of being present: Mindfulness and its role in psychological well-being. *Journal of Personality and Social Psychology, 84,* 822–848.

Haque, A. (1998). Psychology and religion: Their relationship and integration from an Islamic perspeperspective. *American Journal of Islamic Social Sciences, 15*(4), 97–116.

Henry, H. M. (2015). Spiritual energy of Islamic prayers as a catalyst for psychotherapy. *Journal of Relligious Health, 54,* 387–398. https://doi.org/10.1007/s10943-013-9780-4

Hodge, D. R. (2002). Working with Muslim youths: Understanding the values and beliefs of Islamic Islamic discourse. *Children & Schools, 24*(1), 6–20.

Hodge, D. R., & Nadir, A. (2008). Moving toward culturally competent practice with Muslims: Modifying cognitive therapy with Islamic tenets. *Social Work, 53*(1), 31–41. https://doi.org/10.1093/sw/53.1.31

Hoot, J. L., Szecsi, T., & Moosa, S. (2003). What teachers of young children should know about IslamIslam,. *Early Childhood Education Journal, 31*(2), 84–89. https://doi.org/10.1023/B:ECEJ.0000005306.23082.7f

Husain, A. (2006). *Islamic psychology: Emergence of a new field.* Daryaganj, New Delhi: Global Vision.

Inayat, Q. (2005). The Islamic concept of the self. *British Counseling Review, 20,* 2–10.

Jafari, M. F. (1993). Counseling values and objectives: A comparison of Western and Islamic perspectives. *American Journal of Islamic Social Sciences, 10*(3), 326–339.

Keshavarzi, H., & Haque, A. (2013). Outlining a psychotherapy model for enhancing Muslim mental health within an Islamic context. *International Journal for the Psychology of Religion, 23,* 230–249. https://doi.org/10.1080/10508619.2012.712000

Khalili, S., Murken, S., Reich, K. H., Shah, A. A., & Vahabzadeh, A. (2002). Religion and mental health in cultural perspective: Observations and reflections after the first International Congress on Religion and Mental Health, Tehran, April 16–19, 2001. *International Journal for the Psychology of Religion, 12*(4), 217–237.

Mohamed, B. (2016). *A new estimate of the U.S. Muslim population.* http://

www.pewresearch.org/fact-tank/2016/01/06/a-new-estimate-of-the-u-s-muslim-population/

Mohamed, Y. (1986). *The Islamic conception of human nature with special reference to the development development of Islamic psychology.* Unpublished PhD thesis, University of Cape Town.

Mohamed, Y. (1995). *Fitrah and* its bearing on the principles of Islamic psychology. *American Journal of Islamic Social Sciences, 12*(1), 1–18.

Moughrabi, F. (2000). Islam and psychology. In A. E. Kazdin (Ed.), *Encyclopedia of psychology,* vol. 4 pp. 366–368. Washington, DC: American Psychological Association.

Murken, S., & Shah, A. A. (2002). Naturalistic and Islamic approaches to psychology, psychotherapy, and religion: Metaphysical assumptions and methodology—A discussion. *International Journal for the Psychology of Religion, 12*(4), 239–254.

Naeem, F., Gobbi, M., Ayub, M., & Kingdon, D. (2009). University students' views about compatibility of cognitive behavior therapy (CBT) with their personal, social, and religious values (a study from Pakistan). *Mental Health, Religion, & Culture, 12*(8), 847–855. http://dx.doi.org/10.1080/13674670903115226

Pearce, M. J., Robins, C. J., Cohen, H. J., Koenig, H. G., Nelson, B., Shaw, S. F., & King, M. B. (2015). Religiously integrated cognitive behavioral therapy: A new method of treatment for major depression in patients with chronic medical illness. *Psychotherapy, 52*(1), 56–66. https://doi.org/10.1037/a0036448

Piaget, J. (1936). *The origins of intelligence in children.* London: Routledge & Kegan Paul.

Pridmore, S., & Pasha, M. I. (2004). Psychiatry and Islam. *Australasian Psychiatry, 12*(4), 380–385385. https://doi.org/10.1080/j.1440-1665.2004.02131.x.

Qara'ati, M. (2014). *The radiance of the secrets of prayer.* Ahl al-Bayt World Assembly.

Ross-Sheriff, F., & Husain, A. (2004). South Asian Muslim children and families. In R. Fong (Ed.), *Cultturally competent practice with immigrant and refugee children and families,* pp. 163–182). New York: Guilford Press.

Saunders, S. M., Miller, M. L., & Bright, M. M. (2010). Spiritually conscious psychological care. *Professional Psychology: Research and Practice, 41*(5), 355–362. https://doi.org/10.1037/a0020953

Seda, P. (2002). *Islam is . . . : An introduction to Islam and its principles.* Rabwah, Pakistan: Islamic Propagation Propogation Office in Rabwah.

Sheikh, A., & Gatrad, A. R. (2000). *Caring for Muslim patients.* London: Radcliffe Medical Press.

Smither, R., & Khorsandi, A. (2009). The implicit personality theory of Islam. *Psychology of Religion Religion and Spirituality, 1*(2), 81–96. http://dx.doi.org/10.1037/a0015737

Utz, A. (2011). *Psychology from an Islamic perspective*. Olayah, Riyadh, Saudi Arabia: International Islamic Publishing House.

Vahidid-Motlagh, L., & Kajbaf, M. B. (2011). The effectiveness of cognitive behavioral and religious cognitive therapy on anxiety in students. *Journal of Behavioral Sciences*, 5(3), 195–201.

Weatherhead, S., & Daiches, A. (2015). Key issues to consider in therapy with Muslim families. *Journal of Religious Health*, 54, 2398–2411. https://doi.org/10.1007/s10943-015-0023-8

York Al-Karam, C. (2017). *Background paper for CILE seminar*. Center for Islamic Legislation and Ethics seminar on Islamic Psychology, April 2–4, 2018, Doha, Qatar.

CHAPTER 9

Integrating Duaa Arafa and Other Shiite Teachings into Psychotherapy

Sayyed Mohsen Fatemi, PhD

I dedicate this chapter to the dearest soul of my mother, Mahvash Jadali, who just passed away. She was an angel who taught me the art of praying, the art of thinking, and the art of loving.

Any form of therapy is embedded within a specific ontological and epistemological system where modes of knowing and nature of existence are already defined and explicated. Therapists may apply and move in line within what their already established system prescribes or proscribes. Therapists may not necessarily be in touch with the underlying ontological and epistemological components of their therapeutic approach, but as soon as they choose to apply one method or approach over the other, they inevitably follow the guiding principles of the given approach. For instance, as soon as one selects to abide by the psychoanalytical approach in the overall therapeutic process, one ineluctably distances oneself from prescribing the power of prayer as a prescriptive intervention.

In this chapter, I argue that Islamic-based psychology may be positioned within a distinct paradigm with its own productive implications. A spiritually integrated psychotherapy with Muslims may also be placed within this overall holistic Islamic system that operates based on the principles and premises that ultimately share common views and perspectives with the original structural reference points of an Islamic school of thought. I plan to discuss one of so many viable interventions inspired in the heart of an Islamic-based psychology, especially the Shiite perspective.

Spiritually integrated psychotherapy with Muslims requires a solid understanding of the Islamic culture and the Islamic perspective as a leading doctrine with significant prescriptive and proscriptive implications. This would suggest that the religious perspective of Islam, albeit independent, needs to be understood within the cultural situations of clients. This understanding may facilitate the process of accessing a great repertoire of knowledge within the Islamic perspective as a religion that can be reflected in the clients' mode of living. For instance, clients who come from the Muslim world may incorporate *duaa* (prayers) and *dhikr* (recitations of special holy words or verses) in their daily life as a strong source of emotional and spiritual support. It may be very common to see Muslims engage in daily *dhikr* and *duaa*. This is in addition to the daily prayers to be observed five times a day. From an Islamic perspective, *duaa* can have a great impact on improving and transforming one's life. A hadith from Imam Baqer (*salavatollah alayh*), and important Imam in the Shia tradition, indicates that *duaa* or prayer can change one's firmly determined destination. The same Imam was asked whether the virtue of reciting the holy Quran is more than the virtue of praying. The Imam answered that reciting prayer and the act of praying are more preferable. In line with the same understanding, *duaa* and prayers can be applied in psychotherapeutic contexts. This is contrary to the traditional psychoanalytic perspective where spiritual, mystical, and religious experiences were considered signs of pathology or, in Freud's words, "regression to primary narcissism." Numerous studies within psychotherapy have confirmed the positive implications of prayer and contemplative acts in facilitating the process of well-being, or creating helpful psychological treatment interventions (e.g., see Brelsford, 2011; Brelsford & Mahoney, 2002).

I have taught a wide variety of psychotherapeutic approaches, including psychoanalysis, psychodynamics, existential therapy, Gestalt therapy, cognitive behavioral therapy (CBT), dialectical behavioral therapy (DBT), and narrative therapy, and have used them in practice as the occasion required. However, my primary theoretical orientation is with

Langerian mindfulness. Langerian mindfulness is an orientation that helps the client seek novelty and celebrate the phenomenological presence in the moment (see Fatemi, 2016a, b, &c; 2018). There are essentially two different types of mindfulness: meditation-based mindfulness, which is primarily identified with the works by John Cabot Zinn and Langerian mindfulness, characterized by the works of Ellen J. Langer and her long-standing forty-year research findings at Harvard University. Meditation-based mindfulness posits that meditation is the requirement for achieving mindfulness, whereas Langerian mindfulness argues that although meditation can rigorously contribute to the implementation of mindfulness, one may embrace mindfulness without using meditation. In delineating Langerian mindfulness, one is encouraged to explore and seek novelty in any situation, celebrate the possibility of multiple perspectives, live proactively and presently in the moment with a phenomenological engagement, and understand the context and its specific features in different individual, social, cultural, political, economic, psychological, and educational levels (see Fatemi, 2016; 2018).

In dealing with Muslim clients, I have comfortably applied mindfulness in its Islamic context, where the client is released from fragmentation, multiplicities, absence, mindlessness, and estrangement. One of the greatest tools to facilitate the process of this Islamic-based mindfulness happens through the power of prayer, *duaa* and *dhikr*. In Islamic-based mindfulness, presence is the key to empowerment. Presence unfolds itself in directing the attention to God Almighty: Presence entails a liberation. One needs to liberate his or her attention from everything and focus on the real *source* of everything: God. A person who is suffused with attention toward appearance and worldly engagements may experience multiplicity, absence, and mindlessness. In Islamic-based mindfulness, one gains presence through a deliberate attention toward God as the manifestation of all virtues and beauties and the epitome of absolute perfection. To help the client become emancipated from the cognitive and emotional impediments that stand in the way of paying attention to the presence of God serves as a preamble of Islamic-based mindfulness.

In line with different therapeutic schools of thought and their respective therapeutic interventions, such as cognitive therapy, emotion-focused therapy, biological therapies, psychoanalysis, and so on, a wide variety of studies indicate that prayer and religious or mystical experiences have a significant impact in enhancing one's well-being and removing or reducing depression, anxiety, and feelings of hopelessness and helplessness (see, e.g., Levin & Chatters, 2008; Ferraro & Albrecht-Jensen, 1991; Wachholtz & Pargament, 2005, 2008; Spilka, 2003).

In explicating the following case, I try to elucidate that prayer, *duaa*, and dhikr can be suitably applied in dealing with Muslim clients who practice Islam and observe these practices. In particular, I intend to focus on a well-known prayer that is particularly cherished by Shiites called *duaa Arafa*. The prayer was articulated in the plain of Arafa by Imam Husain, the grandson of Prophet Mohammed, the third Imam of Shiites. The prayer has several layers and dimensions, including the monotheistic, educational, ontological, epistemological, and ethical layers. I argue that *duaa Arafa* can also give rise to a very high level of mindfulness, where the client can experience a transcendental sense of awareness with a radical transformation of consciousness. In discussing *duaa* within the context of spiritually integrated psychotherapy, one may delve into the connection between the presence inspired by mindfulness in its Langerian sense and the presence engendered by a sincere and wholehearted connection to God as the source of all blessings and graces.

In doing spiritually integrated psychotherapy with Muslims, additional factors may be included. They are not limited to foundational components of the Islamic perspective as a general interconnected system. They consist of specific terminologies and their associated contextualization, such as *dhikr, duaa, maueza, moraqebah, nafs, towbe,* and so on. For instance, *qalb* (heart) constitutes one of the essential components of Islamic-based psychotherapy, and it consists of so many divisions. *Qalb* is not just referring to the physiological heart but to something quite different. As it is stated in the Quran, there are people who have *qalb* (physiological hearts) but are devoid of *qalb* (the divine and spiritual heart). There are *qalb*s that are locked, and there are enlivened ones. One of the core elements of doing psychotherapy in the Islamic context is to help the client enhance the level of their *qalb*'s receptiveness so that they get empowered to enhance their comprehensive attention toward the ubiquitous presence of God. The therapist helps the clients explore their *qalb* status and expand their level of *qalb*'s elevation through strategies such as *dhikr*. *Dhikr* explicates an ongoing connectedness and remembrance of God. Salavat and *dhikr* open up *qalb* and make it ready to experience the spiritual illumination. *Dhikr* can also be classified in several layers; one is the language-oriented *dhikr* followed by the *qalb*-oriented *dhikr*. Muslim psychotherapists or those dealing with Muslim clients need to be aware of the specific language of the Islamic perspective in dealing with psychological well-being.

Duaa Arafa is one of the well-known key prayers in Islamic doctrine, especially for Shiites. The *duaa* is attributed to Imam Hossein (*salavatollah alayh*), which, according to tradition, has been articulated and recited by Imam Hossein, the third Imam of Shiites (*salavatollah alayh*) on the ninth day of the Arabic month of Zelhajja, known as the day of Arafa in the plain of Arafa. Shiites recite the *duaa* on this day and in the plain of Arafa as well as other mosques in the world. The *duaa* entails numerous spiritual and mystical instructions. Some of the most important features of the *duaa* include:

- ▸ Knowledge toward God and description of God's attributes
- ▸ Pledging with God
- ▸ Knowledge of prophets and reconnecting with them
- ▸ Attention toward the hereafter
- ▸ Purification of the heart and the soul
- ▸ Expressing the infinite blessings of God
- ▸ A journey toward the inner world and the outer world
- ▸ Praising God for the infinite blessings
- ▸ Appealing to God Almighty and expressing repentance and asking for forgiveness
- ▸ Embracing virtues and good deeds
- ▸ Appealing to God Almighty, which begins with *salavat*

Salavat literally means sending greetings to Prophet Mohammed and His Progeny or Household; it asks God to send His blessings and greetings to Prophet Mohammed and His Household. Reciting *salavat* has many implications: It elevates the status of the Prophet and His Household, including the Infallible Imams, so that their level of elevation is continuously upgraded. God is infinite and does not have any limitations, and thus *salavat* brings one closer to God. It is believed that *salavat* helps the reciter experience an existential enhancement so that his or her soul moves toward further enrichment. It is also believed that it removes sins and upgrades the soul. *Duaa* Arafa is also asking for illuminating guidance; blessings; compassion; grace; well-being; health, spiritual, intellectual, emotional, and economic developments; and so on.

In expounding the following example, I demonstrate how *duaa*, especially *duaa Arafa*, can be mindfully introduced in the psychotherapeutic context with a focus on helping clients get over problems with stress, depression, anxiety, and relationship malfunction.

Ahmad came to therapy due to what he described as "debilitating, annihilating, and depreciating quality of life." He was a depressed forty-five-year-old senior manager in a high-tech company with a wife also diagnosed with depression. He was on medication because of his depression. Nonetheless, he was complaining that his medications had not been very effective in helping him cope with his problems. He described his recent days as "gloomy and dismal." His life was dull, stressful, and excruciatingly painful because of highly demanding conditions at work, lack of support from within the family, and an ever-increasing sense of loneliness. He also complained about his relationship with his wife, as her depression had an impact on their communication and especially their sex life. Ahmad described himself as a practicing Muslim but was wondering how he could establish a link between his religious perspective and a solution for dealing with his problems. He came to therapy while wearing a black shirt as a sign to commemorate the martyrdom anniversary of Imam Hossein (*salavatollah alayh*) in the month of Muharram, and he was desperately looking for practical religiously inspired solutions to help him out. The month of Muharram is of great importance for Shiites as it coincides with the martyrdom anniversary of Imam Hossein (*salavatollah alayh*) and his seventy-two followers, who were martyred by Yazid and his soldiers in the day of Ashura. Imam Hossein (*salavatollah alayh*) stood against the tyranny of Yazid and his oppressive regime. Yazid insisted the Imam comply with and give allegiance to Yazid in accepting and endorsing his kingdom and his tyranny against Muslims. The Imam refused and revolted against him, describing Yazid's political and governing style as something that went against the instructions of the holy Prophet Mohammed (*salavatollah alayh va aleh ajmaeen*). In illustrating his mission of revolution, Imam Hossein (*salavatollah alayh*) described his movement as an action to revitalize the prophetic-oriented values and bring livelihood to the Muslim society, which had been darkened and decayed by the demise of human values by Yazid and his regime. Yazid was the son of Moaveehey, who misused the name of Islam to exploit and manipulate Musilm society of the time to proceed with his own utilitarian and materialistic desires. I asked Ahmed the relevance between his beliefs about Imam Hossein and its implications for his well-being. He indicated that his recitation of *duaas* has helped him in the past but nowadays he was overwhelmed by so many things that he hardly even had time to do his daily prayers.

Imam Hossein has a special status among Shiites and is not merely a social or a political leader. The Infallible Imams are known to be the epitome of God on earth. They are known as the perfect human beings with possession of Godly attributes. They are not God but the representatives of God who show the path toward God. Their direction is not separate from God, and they don't claim independence of their own but they are facilitators toward God. They demonstrate in words and action the virtues of a perfect human being, so their words are light and they are the manifestations of God's attributes. Along with their belief in monotheism (*tawheed*), God's Justice (*adl*), the Hereafter and the Day of Resurrection (*ma'ad*), Shiites believe in the leadership of the Infallible Imams (*Imamat*). According to *Imamat*, the Imams are not just social or political leaders who guide people in social contexts, but they can also serve the manifestation of the perfect human being who is close to God in all attributes and features. In Shiites' perspective, Imams are the guiding lights, the illuminating signs, the pillars of truth, and the treasures of the knowledge and wisdom. To abide by Imams in actions would help one elevate one's soul. *Tavassol* is one of the key elements of Shiites: it consists in having attention and taking recourse to the Imams so that they can help people to upgrade themselves. It is stated in the Quran, "O you who believe! Do your duty to Allah and fear Him. Seek the means of approach to Him" (Surat Maideh 35). *Tavassol* has special spiritual and mystical implications among Shiites and can be taken into account as an effective way to achieve wishes, remove difficulties or hardships, or remedy an ailment.

Ahmad, the client, considered himself as very far from a needed spiritual connection due to an immersion in the hackneyed material world. He felt disappointed to the extent that he thought God did not like him. He was also filled with feelings of guilt and blame because of what he described as his inattention to his wife's interests and concerns. I took it upon myself to benefit from his beliefs and connection to Imam Hossein and demonstrate how the Imam's words and wisdom could open up ways of reflection and reflexivity for his surmounting the problems of disappointment, helplessness, and desperation.

Discussion

Ahmed's case can be analyzed in several layers. When stressed out, people usually experience what is called *negative interpretation bias*, where they only look at deficiencies and shortages in life. In order to develop a balance, one needs to be encouraged to see the existing positive features while being exposed to the stressors. This can take place through a variety of empirically proven, effective interventions, including reexamining and reexploring one's perspective. This shift of perspective would occur through a shift of attention to potentially existing windows of opportunities that are usually concealed due to one's mindlessness in one's perspective. In other words, acting from one single emotional and cognitive perspective may not allow the person to experience an alternative mode of perception that would substantiate the power of choices in deciding how to deal with a given situation.

In the Islamic school of thought, plenty of interventions can help out the person under stress. One of the highly recommended strategies is to enliven connection with the transcendental level of life, which encourages one to see and seek meanings beyond the mundane material level. This connection can transpire through reading and being in contact with prayers received from Prophet Mohammed (*salavatollah alayh va aleh*) and or his progeny and the Infallible Imams (*salavatollah alayhem ajmaeen*). *Duaa Arafa* can be well classified into one of the interventions that present multifarious aspects of cognitive, emotional, and behavioral mindfulness within the Islamic perspective.

In part of the *duaa*, the significance of care and nourishment for the soul appears to be vitally important. The care requires attention to the intricate nature of the soul with understanding the essential need for the soul to be connected to a higher realm of being. Ahmad was invited to see that he was not lonely and alone as he could be well connected to the quintessential source of being. I used the analogy of opening the window and experiencing the fresh air. How does the fragrance of the fresh air feel? What does that experience look like? Ahmad was asked to reflect on the questions. I asked him later what happens when he is connected to a source that is ubiquitous and has all blessings, beauties, and graces and is away from any deficiencies and shortages.

I encouraged him to see the implications of the following piece of the prayer: "He is also the Hearer of the prayers, the Warder-off of anguishes, the Raiser of ranks, and the Suppressor of the tyrants." I encouraged him to vividly examine his connectedness to the infinite source of grace and beauty, compassion and blessings. I asked him what would happen if he was constantly connected to the Source with no impediment in the way of the connection. God never sleeps, nor does He take a nap. He never gets tired of listening to us. He knows not only what we say on the surface but is also fully aware of the hidden meanings and intentions beneath what is said. These questions were used to help him probe his monotheistic perspective in illuminating his path with the blessings and the power of hope. The point was not to negate his problems but to indicate that while acknowledging the stressful situations, he could also see the power of his choices to overcome the problem. Instead of his being overwhelmed by the problem, he was encouraged to see that he could own the problem rather than being owned by the problem. In doing so, the perceptiveness toward understanding God as the source of tranquility and composure could be well applied in this case. Again, the point was to help Ahmed reflect on his self-talk. Depression has been associated with cognitive, emotional, and behavioral impairments that can have negative intrapersonal and interpersonal outcomes (see, for instance, Beck, 1967; Feeser et al., 2013; Shiratori et al., 2014; Wilson & Deane, 2010). Notwithstanding the fact that Muslims may observe certain religious rituals and ceremonies, they may not be often vigilant toward the psychological aspects of their practice. In other words, they may not have had the opportunity to reflect on the phenomenological dimensions of their life and their connection to their ontological and epistemological religious outlooks.

I invited Ahmad to reflect on Imam Hossein's words on the day of Ashura before approaching his martyrdom where he addressed God, saying, "You have always been the point of my reliance and hope in the midst of hardships and encumbrances. Many difficult situations that weakened the number of friends and amassed the number of enemies, and You did not leave me alone and you provided me with support and care."

The point was to help him understand what his role model, Prophet Mohammed, would have done in a similar situation. This reflective journey tended to explicate the point of distancing him from his situation and problems so that he could see that despite his entanglements, he could separate himself from his problems.

Ahmad was encouraged to understand the distinction between identifying himself with the depression, negativity, anxiety, helplessness, fear, and so on, and deconstructing them from him. When depression reigns over one's thoughts, feelings, and behaviors, one is exposed to a fallacy that he or she *is* the depression. Ahmad was invited to reflect on the implications of the prayer in attesting to negating all possessiveness clouded in the pseudo-manifestation of ego. Ego brings the falsehood of sensibility by relying on itself, by attributing everything to its sovereignty and power. The prayer reiterates that egoism and egotism are mirages of power. They do not exist at all in the real ontological taxonomy of existence. They are pretentious and ostentatious simulacrum that do not carry any authenticity. The interpretive contextual layers of *duaa* helped Ahmad to see how his life had been associated with so many subjective dimensions of his socially constructed world. He further realized that through an indulgence in the material world, he had distanced from an in-depth examination of his connectedness to a bigger realm of existence. This was not meant to downgrade the significance of his daily problems at work but to highlight the vitality of his mindful agency, namely his power of choices to overcome problems instead of passively escaping from responsibility.

In an Islamic context, mindfulness unfolds its power in a lively phenomenological connection to the presence of God. God is closer to one than anything else. It is stated in the Quran, "It was We who created man, and We know what dark suggestions his soul makes to him: for We are nearer to him than [his] jugular vein" (Surah Qaf 16). Ahmad was invited to explore his intrapersonal mindfulness to the effect that he understood his internal source of security. This helped him realize what served as his commanding center of security. I explained to him the difference between the importance of things and their being changed into a commanding center. On the positive side, wealth, money, power, reputation, financial success, and so forth can be important things to acquire, but if they turn out to be the commanding center of one's life, they would take over one's security; when they are present, the person would feel secure and safe, and when they go away, one's vulnerability would emerge. This would lead to mindlessness in an Islamic context in that one would move toward a direction that stands in opposition to his or her well-being and health. On the negative side, too, sorrow, sadness, and desperation could be taken as the essential features of the material world, but if they occupy one's soul and take over one's command of life, one would experience a departure from his or her true presence, thus disconnecting from the real source of presence: God. In *duaa Arafa*, one learns to constantly remind oneself not to be forgetful of the presence of God, as He can unlock any locks and knots.

Ahmad continued his counseling sessions and was able to increase his level of religious mindfulness through reciting *dhikr* and *salavat* (may Allah's blessings beam on Prophet Mohammed and his progeny), which he believed helped him in the past, too. Like meditation-based mindfulness and its focus on a mantra or breathing, the Islamic school of thought has an emphasis on reciting *salavat*. *Salavat*, according to numerous hadiths, has a healing impact in which the person would upgrade his or her soul. Imam Reza (*salavatollah alayh*) indicates that *salavat* dissipates the sins. Ahmad's recitation and reflection on the implications of *duaa*, especially his reflection on the meanings of *duaa Arafa*, facilitated the process of distancing him from the problems and detaching from stressful situations. He was also able to broaden his perspective and pay attention to his wife's interests and concerns. This came out of his revisiting his interpersonal relationship through a more rigorous focus on *duaa Arafa* and its implications for relationship betterment. His eyes filled with tears when we discussed a hadith from Imam Hossein (*salavatolah alayh*). The hadith described that one day Imam Hossein was having a loaf of bread while a dog was lying in front of him. The Imam gave half of the loaf to the dog before having a loaf of his own. A witness asked Imam if it was okay to let the dog go hungry, and the Imam warned the person against doing so by saying, "I would be ashamed to be indifferent toward a creature of God in front of me" (see Hakimi, 2004). The question for Ahmad here was when our role model is so meticulously mindful and sensitive toward the rights of animals, how could he ever be so cruel against his wife's rights and presence? As for his feelings of guilt and self-blame, Ahmad elicited from the spirit of the prayer and came to realize the possibility of having hopes and experiencing compassion and forgiveness. *Duaa Arafa* taught him to understand that despair is to turn your back on God, and one who despairs and experiences despondency is getting further from God. As such, a fatal mistake is to experience despair and hopelessness.

Conclusion

Doing spiritually integrated psychotherapy with Muslims is so delicately interwoven with so many subtle layers. One of the significant dimensions of doing Islamic-based therapy with Muslims lies in a recondite understanding of Islam and its principles. In addition, the therapist needs to be familiar with the cultural contexts and subcontexts. Understanding the underlying elements of the clients' affective, associative, and marginal meanings and their embodiments in their cultural configuration would help the therapist apply the right techniques in different contexts.

Imam Sadeq (*salavatollah alayh*), enumerating the conditions of effective communication for conveying the message of Islam, underlines that one needs to discuss and apply what is already familiar to clients and not apply or discuss what is unfamiliar to them. In another hadith, Imam Ali (*salavatollah alayh*) presents an effective communication skill by saying we should talk to people based on their capacities, competencies, and intelligence (see Hakimi, 2004).

One cannot forbear adding that a well-versed therapist with an erudition on different Western systems of psychotherapy needs to select integrative approaches in dealing with Muslim clients, but in order to do Islamic-based psychotherapy, the therapist needs to have a great and in-depth understanding of the Islamic school of thought and its ontological and epistemological layers. This also includes a comprehensive perceptiveness of hadiths and their application and implications in a wide variety of contexts.

References

Beck A. T. (1967). Depression: *Clinical, experimental, and theoretical aspects.* New York: Hoeber.

Brelsford, G. M. (2011). Divine alliances to handle family conflict: Theistic meditation and triangulation in father-child relationships. *Psychology of Religion and Spirituality, 3,* 285–297.

Brelsford, G. M., & Mahoney, A. (2008). Spiritual disclosure between older adolescents and their mothers. *Journal of Family Psychology, 22,* 62–70.

Fatemi, S. M. (2014). Exemplifying a shift of paradigm: Exploring the psychology of possibility and embracing the instability of knowing. In A. I., C. T. Ngnoumen, & E. J. Langer (Eds.), *The Wiley Blackwell Handbook of Mindfulness* (pp. 115–138). Malden, MA: John Wiley & Sons.

Fatemi, S. M. (2016a). *Critical mindfulness: Exploring Langerian models.* New York: Springer.

Fatemi, S. M. (2016b). Mindfulness and perceived control: Controlling the impossibility of controllability. In J. W. Reich & F. J. Infurna (Eds.), *Perceived control: Theory, research, and practice in the first 50 years* (pp. 131–146). New York: Oxford University Press.

Fatemi, S. M. (2016c). Langerian mindfulness and liminal performing spaces. In A.

L. Baltzell (Ed.), *Mindfulness and performance* (Current Perspectives in Social and Behavioral Sciences, pp. 112–124). New York: Cambridge University Press.

Fatemi, S. M. (2018). *The psychological power of language*. New York: Routledge.

Fatemi, S. M., & Langer, E. J. (2018). Langerian mindfulness and its psychotherapeutic implications: Recomposing/decomposing mindlessly constructed life stories. In B. Kirkcaldy (Ed.), *Psychotherapy, literature and the visual and performing arts*. London: Palgrave Macmillan.

Fatemi, M., Ward, E. D., and Langer, E. J. (2016). Peak performance: Langerian mindfulness and flow. In A. L. Baltzell (Ed.), Mindfulness and performance (Current Perspectives in *Social and Behavioral Sciences*, pp. 101–111). New York: Cambridge University Press.

Feeser, M., Schlagenhauf, F., Sterzer P., et al. (2013). Context insensitivity during positive and negative emotional expectancy in depression assessed with functional magnetic resonance imaging. *Psychiatry Research: Neuroimaging, 212*, 28–35.

Ferraro, K., & Albrecht-Jensen, C. (1991). Does religion influence adult health? *Journal for the Scientific Study of Religion, 30*(2), 193–202.

Freud, S. (1961). *Civilizations and its discontents*. New York: Norton.

Hakimi, M. R. (2004). *Elaheeyate Elahee va elaheeyate basharee* [Islamic theology and man driven theology]. Daleele Ma Publication. Qom: Iran.

Levin, J., & Chatters, L. M. (2008). Religion, aging, and health: Historical perspectives, current trends, and future directions—public health. *Journal of Religion, Spirituality & Aging, 20*(1), 153–172.

Qomi, S. A. (2011). *Doaa Arafat of Imam Husein*. Compiled in the collection of Mafatihol Jenah [The keys to paradise]. Ajvad Publication. Qom: Iran.

Shiratori, Y., Tachikawa, H., Nemoto, K., Endo, G., Aiba, M., Matsui, Y., & Asada, T. (2014). Network analysis for motives in suicide cases: A cross-sectional study. *Psychiatry and Clinical Neuroscience, 68*(4), 299–307.

Spilka, B. (2003). *The psychology of religion: An empirical approach*. New York: Guilford.

Sundararajan, L., & Fatemi, S. M. (2016). Creativity and symmetry restoration: Toward a cognitive account of mindfulness. *Journal of Theoretical and Philosophical Psychology, 36*(3), 131–141. dx.doi.org/10.1037/teo0000027

Wachholtz, A., & Pargament, K. (2005). Is spirituality a critical ingredient of meditation? Comparing the effects of spiritual meditation, secular meditation, and relaxation on spiritual, psychological, cardiac, and pain outcomes. *Journal of Behavioral Medicine, 28*(4), 369–384.

Wilson, C. J., & Deane, F. P. (2010). Help negation and suicidal ideation: The role of depression, anxiety, and hopelessness. *Journal of Youth and Adolescence, 39*(3), 291–305.

About the Contributors

Layla Asamarai, PsyD, is a licensed psychologist and approved eye movement desensitization and reprocessing (EMDR) consultant. She is currently working at Ramsey County, Minnesota, as a senior clinical psychologist and is the founder and owner of Luminous Mind Inc. She possesses a clinical background that highlights experience in policy change, program development and working with communities of color, survivors of torture, and individuals that struggle with complex and generational trauma. Her experience began in Minneapolis, Minnesota and was followed by eight years of clinical work in Dubai, UAE. In 2016 she returned to serve her community in the Twin Cities Metro Area of Minnesota. In addition to direct service to clients and their families, she enjoys teaching, consultation, and program development.

Sayyed Mohsen Fatemi, PhD, completed his post-doctoral studies in the Department of Psychology at Harvard University, where he also served as a teaching fellow, an associate, and a fellow. He works on mindfulness and its psychological implications for cross-cultural, clinical, and social psychology. He is the author of numerous books and has had articles published in journals, such as the American Psychological Association's *Journal of Theoretical and Philosophical Psychology*. His works have already been published by Springer, Wiley, Cambridge University Press, Oxford University Press, and Palgrave Macmillan. His new book, *The Psychological Power of Language*, was recently published by Routledge. He has two forthcoming books with Routledge and PalgraveMacmillan.

AFSHANA HAQUE, PhD, LMFT-S is a licensed marriage and family therapist supervisor with a specialization in neurofeedback. She is also an assistant professor of marriage and family therapy at the University of Houston–Clear Lake. Dr. Haque earned her PhD from St. Mary's University in San Antonio, Texas. In 2008 she received extensive training in cultural competency as a fellow in the Substance Abuse and Mental Health Services Administration (SAMHSA) American Association of Marriage and Family Therapy (AAMFT) Minority Fellowship Program. Her research interests include the sociopolitical influence on the mental health and well-being of Muslim families, validating relational assessments for use with Muslim populations, and creating therapy models that are palatable to clients from minority and collectivistic cultures. She has published multiple peer-reviewed articles in prestigious journals in her field; she is also a contributing author for Muslim Matters' *What's the Matter?* forum and Stones to Bridges' *Dear Fatima* column. Dr. Haque helped establish and served as a board member for the Center of Refugee Services in San Antonio. She has conducted parenting workshops in the Greater Houston and Austin areas and has presented in both national and international professional conferences. She has also presented in Islamic conferences including ISNA: Islam in America, Texas Dawa Convention, and CAIR. Dr. Haque has been a practicing therapist for about ten years and is the director of her private practice, Muslim Family Support, where she conducts face-to-face and online therapy. She provides hope and relief to clients who present with relational issues around marriage, sex, trauma, addiction, parenting, adolescence, anxiety, depression, spiritual crisis, decreased self-esteem, multicultural relationships, premarital therapy, divorce, and discernment therapy. Dr. Haque takes a collaborative and solution-focused approach when working with clients in therapy.

PAUL M. KAPLICK holds a BSc in applied psychology with a specialization in clinical psychology, and is currently pursuing his graduate studies in the area of brain and cognitive sciences at the Institute for Interdisciplinary Studies at the University of Amsterdam, Netherlands.

He established and heads the Islam and Psychology research group at the Islamic Association of Social and Educational Professions in Frankfurt and Munich, Germany; is a research affiliate of the Muslims and Mental Health Laboratory of Dr. Rania Awaad at Stanford University, Department of Psychiatry and Behavioral Sciences; is a research assistant in the Al-Karam Lab for Islamic Psychology of Dr. Carrie York Al-Karam at the University of Iowa; and has worked at the Institute of Muslim Mental Health under Dr. Hamada Hamid, DO. As an undergraduate, he conducted research at Oxford University (Department of Psychiatry), the Max Planck Institute of Psychiatry in Munich, the Institute for Therapeutic Research Munich, and the Clinic of Psychiatry and Psychotherapy of the Ludwig-Maximilian University Munich.

HOOMAN KESHAVARZI is a licensed psychotherapist in Illinois, completed his PsyD (to be conferred), holds a master's of clinical psychology and a bachelor's of science, specialist psychology track / minor in Islamic studies. He is the founder and executive director of Khalil Center, a mental health institute specializing in the practice of Islamically Integrated psychotherapy and the largest provider of Muslim mental healthcare in the United States. He is also an adjunct professor of psychology at Argosy University Chicago, American Islamic College, and Hartford Seminary, and an instructor of psychology for Islamic Online University. He is a Fellow at the Institute for Social Policy and Understanding at the Global Health Center, conducting research on topics related to Muslims and mental health. Hooman is a national public speaker and trainer currently serving as a clinical supervisor of graduate students of clinical psychology at the Village of Hoffman Estates (DHS). In addition to his academic training, he has studied Islamic theology both formally and informally with a number of Islamic scholars. He was recently appointed Visiting Scholar at Ibn Haldun University in Turkey.

FAHAD KHAN, PsyD, has a doctorate in clinical psychology and a master's degree in biomedical sciences. He is also a Hafiz of the Quran (having committed the entire Quran to memory) and has studied Islam with various scholars in the Muslim world and the U.S. He is currently a student at Darul Qasim continuing his Arabic and Islamic studies under the supervision of Sh. Amin Kholwadia. He is a faculty member at Concordia University Chicago and College of DuPage. He conducts research related to Muslim mental health on topics such as help-seeking attitudes of Muslim Americans, effects of acculturation and religiosity on psychological distress, and other clinically relevant issues. The primary focus of his clinical training has been with children and adolescents suffering from serious mental illnesses. However, he has had a broad range of experience dealing with individuals from all age groups and cultural backgrounds.

FARAH LODI, MA, CCC, is the owner of Moving Forward, a counseling service in Dubai, UAE. Farah has lived on three continents, is multiculturally sensitive, and helps clients from diverse backgrounds in both individual and couples counseling. She has a master's degree in mental health counseling from Seton Hall University in the United States, and is a Canadian-Certified Counselor. She has been a featured writer for the Canadian Counseling and Psychotherapy Association online journal, *Counseling Connect*, and has created an online counseling forum, Support Seekers (www.supportseekers.info), which is a free community service. She is also an adjunct instructor at Zayed University in Dubai, where she supervises psychology interns and is frequently invited as a guest speaker, both in the United Arab Emirates and internationally. In October 2016 she presented a paper on spiritual modeling based on Prophet Mohammed at the International Psychology Conference in Dubai, and was invited to present at the Middle East Psychology Association annual meeting in April 2017. Over the past ten years, she has participated in a study circle focusing on the works of theologians such as Al Ghazali, and through this process developed a special interest in Prophet Mohammed's life. Her recent research focuses on the psychospiritual significance of meditation, especially relating to the ninety-nine names of Allah, and on a psychological analysis of the Prophet Mohammed's resiliency.

RABIA MALIK, PhD, is a consultant systemic psychotherapist. She is a registered practitioner with the United Kingdom Council of Psychotherapists. She teaches part time on the systemic doctorate at the Tavistock Centre in London and runs a part time private practice. She has provided trainings and presented at conferences nationally and internationally on developing cross-cultural therapeutic practice as well as Islamic counselling. Her main interest is in developing therapeutic ways of working with Muslim clients, integrating cultural, religious, and spiritual beliefs with therapeutic practice. She has extensive experience in working with Muslim clients and community organizations. She works with statutory and community organizations on complex cases, including cases involving radicalization. Rabia previously was colead of the Marlborough Cultural Therapy Centre, a specialist service for minority ethnic clients based in a London Natural health Service child and adolescent mental health clinic. She also taught at the University of East London in psychosocial studies. Her doctorate was on the cultural construction of depression among Pakistanis. She has numerous publications based on her work.

ABDALLAH ROTHMAN is a licensed professional counselor (LPC) with fifteen years of experience as a psychotherapist and currently resides in the United Arab Emirates. He holds a master's in psychology and is a doctoral candidate in psychology at Kingston University London. In addition to his academic and clinical training in Western psychology, Abdallah studies and practices Islamic psychology with leaders in the field in the United States, Sudan, Turkey, United Arab Emirates, and the United Kingdom He was an adjunct faculty member at George Washington University, and he established Shifaa Integrative Counseling, a private practice offering Islamically integrated psychotherapy to the Muslim community in Washington, DC Abdallah's clinical practice as well as his academic research focus is on approaching psychotherapy from within an Islamic paradigm and establishing an indigenous Islamic theoretical orientation to human psychology that is grounded in the knowledge of the soul from the Quran and *sunnah.*

IBRAHIM RÜSCHOFF, MD, studied education and medicine in Hamburg and Münster, Germany. He specialized in neurology, psychiatry, and psychotherapy (psychodynamic therapy) and worked as a senior consultant for several hospitals in Germany. Since 2007, he has worked as a licensed medical psychotherapist in a private practice together with his wife, Malika Laabdallaoui. For over thirty-five years, his area of expertise has been the psychosocial support of Muslims in Germany, and he has published several books, book chapters, and journal articles on spiritually integrated psychotherapy with Muslims. He is a member of the German Association for Psychiatry, Psychotherapy and Psychosomatics (DGPPN) and the German Council of Muslims in Germany (ZMD), and he founded the Islamic Association of Social and Educational Professions in Germany in 1989.

DR. FYEQA SHEIKH, PsyD, is a licensed clinical psychologist practicing at Swedish Covenant Hospital in Chicago. She received her doctorate in psychology (PsyD) from the Chicago School of Professional Psychology in 2012, specializing in child and adolescent psychology. Dr. Sheikh's clinical and research interests include South Asian mental health, Islamic psychology, multicultural psychology, utilizing cognitive behavioral techniques to treat depression and anxiety, and trauma-informed treatment. She was afforded the opportunity to participate in the Minority Fellowship Program through the American Psychological Association for her research with Pakistani Muslim American women. Additionally she served on the executive board of the Division on South Asian Americans within the Asian American Psychological Association. She has a strong interest in integrating Islamic principles into psychotherapy and strives to erase the stigma associated with mental health in the Muslim community. In efforts to further this interest, she has coauthored a chapter on Islamic healing in an edited book titled *Multicultural Approaches to Health and Wellness in America*. She also presented clinical applications of Islamic psychology at the ninth annual Muslim Mental Health

Conference. Dr. Sheikh is involved in her community mosque, where she delivers psychologically oriented presentations to parents and the community at large. In addition to her clinical practice and community engagement, she serves as an adjunct faculty member in the Counseling Psychology program at the Chicago School of Professional Psychology.

Index

magic. *See sihr*
mantra repetition, 92
Marcella, A., 7–8
marginalized populations, CRT and, 104
ma'rifa (gnosis), 48
marital counseling, Islamically-guided, 15. *See also* case examples, Islamically integrated family therapy; vignettes, marital counseling
   childhood experiences and, 69
   imams and, 61–62
   Muslim client distrust of, 57–58
   partiality and, 73
   power of, 72–73
   resistance to, 59
Marlborough Family Service, 153
marriage. *See also* vignettes, marital counseling
   affection in, 63
   case examples on sex and, 117–19
   fear of infidelity, 69–71
   financial disputes, between spouses, 65–67, 114–16
   financial disputes in, 65–67, 114–16
   loyalty and infidelity in, 67–71
   Mohammed on, 58
   multicultural/multiracial, 123–24
   spousal roles in, 114–16
   spouse disinterest in sex and intimacy, 62–64
Masjid Al-Haram, 111
Maslow, Abraham, 28
Mecca, 86
meditation, 48–49. *See also* mindfulness; *muraqaba*
   focused (*zikr*), 93
   PTSD and, 94
   talking to God through, 92–93
mental health professionals (MHPs)
   challenges for, 124–25

   collaborative language systems and, 103
   culturally responsive therapy and, 103–5
   non-Muslim, 17
   recommendations and future directions for, 125–26
mental health services
   stigma surrounding seeking of, 9–10, 11, 17–18, 59–60
   suggestions for increasing use of, 224–25
mental illness, 60
MER. *See* Muslim Experiential Religiousness
MHPs. *See* mental health professionals
Michael of East Jane, 169
migrants, children of, 160
mind, overidentifying with, 36
mindfulness, 92, 222, 232
   Islamic-based, 231, 239
misogyny, 66
MMH. *See* Muslim Mental Health
modernity, Islam and, 12
Mohammed (Prophet) (RasoolAl-lah). *See also* hadiths
   Abu Sufyan and, 95, 96
   Cave Thawr incident, 82
   on comparing to others, 113
   compassion after banishment from Mecca, 86
   first wife of, 63, 66, 67
   forgiveness exemplified by, 95
   on gentleness, 67
   on getting treatment, 60
   grandson of, 232
   gratitude exemplified by, 97–98
   Isra Al-Miraj event of, 90
   know thy self words of, 19
   on marriage, 58
   negative emotions and, 79–80